THE STORY OF FIRST KIDNEY TRANSPLANT IN GUYANA, SOUTH AMERICA

THE STORY OF FIRST KIDNEY TRANSPLANT IN GUYANA, SOUTH AMERICA

And Lessons for Developing Countries

Transplant Surgeon, The Walter Reed Army
Medical Center, Washington, DC
Consultant, Systems Assessment and
Research Inc., Lanham, MD
General Surgeon, The Brookdale University
Hospital and Medical Center, Brooklyn, N.Y.
Clinical Professor, The George Washington
University, Washington, D.C.

Rahul M. Jindal, MD, PhD

iUniverse, Inc.
New York   Bloomington

iUniverse books may be ordered through booksellers or by contacting:

iUniverse
1663 Liberty Drive
Bloomington, IN 47403
www.iuniverse.com
1-800-Authors (1-800-288-4677)

Because of the dynamic nature of the Internet, any Web addresses or links
contained in this book may have changed since publication and may no longer be
valid. The views expressed in this work are solely those of the author and do not
necessarily reflect the views of the publisher, and the publisher hereby disclaims
any responsibility for them.

ISBN: 978-1-4401-7387-5 (sc)
ISBN: 978-1-4401-7388-2 (ebook)

Library of Congress Control Number: 2009910862

Printed in the United States of America

iUniverse rev. date: 11/04/09

Also By The Author

The Struggle for Life
Psychological Perspective of Kidney Disease and Transplantation.
Lyndsay S. Baines, Rahul M. Jindal
ISBN: 0-86569-323-4
ISBN-13: 978-0-86569-323-4
Praeger Publishers
Publication: 12/30/2003
Description:

With case examples and step-by-step frameworks for intervention, the authors illustrate the challenges and solutions in establishing an effective ward-based psychotherapy service for renal dialysis and transplant patients. They describe clinical patterns of presentation and how psychotherapeutic intervention was refined over time in a clinically meaningful and evidence-based manner. Each chapter is focused on specific emotional disorders among renal patients.

The authors introduce the concept of loss of an imagined past' (aspirations and ambitions) never realized, or compromised, as a result of renal disease and as a major cause of post-transplant depression. Emotional issues which have received little prior attention in the literature—including substance abuse, eating disorders, gender disorders and emotional body image—are addressed in depth. Practical advice, including that against referencing the transplanted organ as a gift, is offered.

Dedication

This book is dedicated to young Munesh Mangal, to his mother, Ms Leelkumarie Mangal, of Lot 119 Lusignan Pasture, East Coast Demerara, Guyana, and to all kidney failure patients awaiting kidney transplantation.

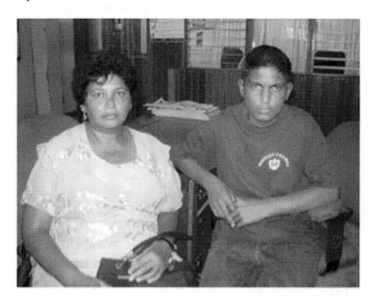

Contents

PROLOGUE

Preface

The book consists of three parts.

The first part of the book narrates the story of a single mother from Georgetown in Guyana who made an appeal to help her son dying of kidney failure to obtain a kidney transplant, which was not available in their country. They needed help to travel to India and get the transplant. The flyer appealing for help lands in the hands of a Guyanese-American, George Subraj, who is intrigued by this appeal. George seeks the help of Rahul M. Jindal, who in turn organizes a medical team. The medical team motivates the local Guyanese physicians and travels to Georgetown to carry out the first kidney transplant in Guyana. This is also a story of how Americans come together to save the life of a young man in Guyana, whose determined single mother refused to give up.

In the second half of the book, we discuss the social aspects of transplantation, which include medical compliance, anxiety and depression in kidney transplant recipients and social networks pertaining to kidney transplantation.

In the third part of the book, we discuss economics of kidney transplantation in developing countries, economics of peritoneal dialysis versus hemodialysis, pre-emptive kidney transplantation for developing countries, health policy for treating renal failure in developing countries and finally commercialization of kidney transplantation—a problem which is increasing world-wide.

Above all, this is a story of the humanity and kindness of American and Guyanese professionals and citizens who gave up their time to make a difference in the life of a young man in Guyana who needed a kidney transplant.

RM Jindal, MD, PhD, MBA
Washington, DC
May 2009

PART 1

Chapter 1:

A Flyer Lands in Queens, New York City

George Subraj is a man of action and of few words, owner of Zara Realty[1], and known as a humanitarian by friends but a slum landlord by his many enemies. George as is known to be flamboyant, always in a suit, tie and a hat—reminds you of a long-gone British era. George likes to eat Indian food, curries and pakoras—but his favorite is shrimp curry accompanied by Yellow Tail wine[2], named after the yellow-footed rock wallaby, a smaller cousin of the kangaroo that has a golden tail. The curry has to be made and eaten at the Royal Indian Palace & Restaurant[3] at the cross roads of Atlantic Avenue and Lefferts Boulevard. George is an American of Guyanese origin, having left Guyana when he was eighteen years old to make a living in the new world and escape the political oppression in Guyana at that time.

George Subraj is at the top of his game. His company is based in Queens, one of the most vibrant and culturally diverse communities in New York, and the neighboring suburb of Nassau County, Long Island. A competitively priced real estate and rental market, coupled with transport orientated development, in the form of Jamaica Station, expedient subway access to Manhattan, two major international airports, JFK adjacent to Jamaica Bay and LaGuardia by the East River, has helped Queens emerge as a bustling heart of commerce, trade and community living. The development of corporate space continues at a rapid pace as does the necessary supportive infrastructure for corporate visitors, the academic community from centers of excellence such as CUNY Law

1   www.zararealty.com
2   http://discoveryellowtail.com/#/home/
3   Royal Indian Palace & Restaurant, 118-08 Atlantic Ave, New York, NY 11419, (718) 846-7600

School and tourists on the ancestral trails of jazz icons such as, Louis Armstrong and Ella Fitzgerald, or the Kaufman studios in Astoria, Shea Stadium and much more. Major hotel chains such as Ramada and Comfort Inn recently opened their doors along with white tablecloth restaurants. While the development of a lush new Green Gateway at downtown town Jamaica's western entrance is imminent and the Jamaica pathways provide green, safe links for pedestrians between parking and commercial areas.

George is meeting with his friends at the Indian restaurant for his usual darbar[4]. The group includes myself, Jaskaran Persaud, and Lakeram Persaud. It is wet and cold, middle of winter in 2008. We order a bottle of Yellow Tail wine, which is our usual. The waiters all know us—including the jovial owner—a Sikh from India, a self made man who is a community leader in Queens. We order shrimp curry, pakoras, rice pullow and lots of yellow dal. As I am vegetarian, I order paneer makhani and green salad. We were talking about how to play the markets and make money and if investing in property was worth it. I asked George "should I invest in the market, mutual funds or stock or a building?" George in his usual wise mind says "buy a building or land only if can manage it and have hands on approach". We talk a bit more on money markets and politics of his native Guyana and I was telling them of my recent visit to see my folks in Ahmedabad, India[5].

George in the middle of this fine dinner meeting pulls out a print out of an appeal:

Friday, January 4, 2008
Mom Pleads for Kidney Transplant to Save Son's Life[6]
Below is a story I noticed this evening in the Guyana Chronicle about a young man with "end stage renal failure" and his mother's plea for help. The single mother is giving her kidney to her son, but needs monetary help to pay for his kidney transplant. This story struck a personal chord with me because my grandmother passed away more than a year ago from complications related to kidney failure and she

4   A term for a court in Urdu from the Persian - Durbar (court).
5   http://www.thebestofindia.com/City/ahmedabad.asp
6   http://www.caribvoice.org/Pop%20Ups/help.html

underwent painful dialysis prior to her death. Believe me, it's a hellish experience for a family to go through. Fortunately, she lived a long life, but this young man won't if he doesn't get help soon. I hope there's a doctor out there reading this story who can sponsor this surgery.

LEELKUMARIE Mangal, 41, of Lot 119 Lusignan Pasture, East Coast Demerara, is appealing to the business community and the general public to help her son get a kidney transplant in India and dialysis treatment here. She said her son, Munesh Mangal, 18, was diagnosed with 'end stage renal failure' in August last year, after he became ill and was a patient for two months at Georgetown Public Hospital Corporation (GPHC).

The woman told the Guyana Chronicle yesterday that he currently receives haemodialysis treatment at 5G Dialysis Centre, Lots 235-236 Baramita and Aubrey Barker Streets, South Ruimveldt, Georgetown, at a cost of G$100,000 weekly.

"I cannot afford to meet that amount so often and this is why I am asking for help to raise the funds," she appealed.

It is very difficult for him to cope and is often overwhelmed with pain and the burden of long-term dialysis treatment would be impossible for her to meet as a single parent, his mother said.

She said she is willing to donate one of her kidneys for the operation in India but has to raise US$36,000 for expenses.

Munesh said he was forced to leave the private school he attended when he took sick suddenly.

Persons willing to contribute to his cause can do so through Guyana Bank for Trade and Industry (GBTI) account SIEA 753156.

His mother, a vendor of green vegetables, said she approached the Ministry of Health and was assisted with the payment for 10 dialysis treatments which he has already received.

She can be reached on telephone numbers 220-_ _ _ _, 646- _ _ _ _, and 653-_ _ _ _. (Michel Outridge)

George asks me "doc what do you think of this?"

"I am a Transplant Surgeon; it is a straight forward operation in the US and many countries in the world, it is done in at least eight centers in New York City."

I get these questions all the time as friends, colleagues, waiters in restaurants, and shop owners try to get curbside consults[7] when they find out that I am a Transplant Surgeon. I love doing curbside consults, except when I am enjoying a good Indian dinner at our favorite restaurant. Also, it was suggested that curbside consults could lead to malpractice suits, a practice that has been a matter of much debate and controversy[8]. However, most physicians take this in their stride.

George was more curious as he read the piece of paper again: "What does it cost?"

"Something in the region of 100,000 dollars, depending on the center, insurance carrier, and cost of medications."

George was even more curious "What are the complications of surgery. What is the cost of medications?"

I gave him the run down on a laundry list of complications, side effects of medications, and need for life-long follow up with specialists.

We finish the dinner, walk out to our cars and go back to our houses.

---

7   Washington School of Medicine: Risk Prevention and Control: Informal "Curbside" Consultations. http://aladdin.wustl.edu/risk/riskmgmt.nsf/00e6edf0d1cc3393862567f50051bbd9/2ab531e88d4ce3698625 67f5005e36f9?OpenDocument

8   http://www.curbsideconsult.org/

Chapter 2:
George Calls Rahul Jindal

I got a call from George Subraj on February 6, 2008, asking me to join him at our favorite restaurant in Queens. I asked him what the occasion was—a birthday or some anniversary? "No, just come and we will have a good Indian dinner"

I was finishing my work at the Brookdale University Hospital and Medical Center[9], where I am an Attending Surgeon. Brookdale University Hospital and Medical Center is a very hectic place, busy trauma center, but with a caring staff. It caters to some of the most deprived zones of New York City. The Department of Surgery is headed by a distinguished senior Surgeon, Dr. Richard Fogler, MD, FACS. Dr. Folger is like a father figure to many of the residents and faculty. Most of the surgical faculty had been at this hospital for many years, having served as residents and progressed to faculty. Also, I was in the process of relocating to Walter Reed Army Medical Center[10], a fine national institution for the Department of Defense. They have the only transplant program for the Department of Defense.

The Royal Punjab restaurant is only 6 miles from Brookdale University Hospital and Medical Center; however parking is an issue as the restaurant is right at the junction of Atlantic Avenue and Lefferts Boulevard. So I suggested to George Subraj that we meet somewhere else, perhaps the Indian Heritage in Long Island[11], which has more parking space and also serves really classic Indian food. However, George Subraj insists on meeting at The Royal Punjab as he is craving for his favorite shrimp curry and Yellow Tail wine. We meet at about

9   http://www.brookdale.edu/
10   http://www.wramc.army.mil/support/Pages/default.aspx
11   http://www.heritageindiancuisine.com/

5:00 PM, a time which George Subraj insists on, I prefer a later time for dinner. Anyway, George Subraj is waiting for me at the restaurant with wine in his hands. Also, in the group are Jaskaran Persuad and Lakeram Persaud. George was bubbling with enthusiasm and energy. I assumed that he made another kill in the property market—perhaps beat someone else to acquiring another apartment block. I was wrong.

George "Rahul, have you visited Guyana?"

"No, what's there to see in Guyana?"

George "Guyana has the Kaieteur Falls[12,] want to come and see the famous Falls?"

"Not really, I am setting up a practice and there is too much to do at the hospital. Besides, it's a long way to see the Kaieteur Falls."

George "Guyana is also becoming popular with tourists for the rain forest, in fact, eco-tourism is the fastest growing economic sectors in Guyana."

George "If you wish to come, we will buy the tickets and get you to see not only Kaieteur Falls, but also Georgetown Public Hospital[13.]"

"Why would I want to fly 5 hours to see a public hospital in a relatively poor country with ethnic problems[14,] and besides I don't have a Guyanese visa."

George "You don't require visa if you have US citizenship and anyway, I already have the airline tickets."

"Good for you have fun."

George "Yes, we will have fun, we will be staying at the famous Buddy's International Hotel[15.]"

"We?"

It then suddenly connected—the pieces of the puzzle, the flyer, the appeal of a mother for her son's kidney transplant, the invitation for dinner and the "we".

"George, I don't know—I may be on call and I really don't like long flights, I get jet-lag."

---

12 http://www.kaieteurpark.gov.gy/

13 http://www.hospitalsworldwide.com/listings/14732.php (New Market Street, Georgetown, Guyana, Tel: 227-8232/8204-9 or +592 2 5690, Additional Information: 600 beds - main referral hospital in Guyana)

14 http://www.coha.org/2004/07/guyana-born-a-broken-nation-always-a-broken-nation/

15 http://www.buddysguyana.com/

"Besides, is it safe? I heard about the Jonestown massacre of Jim Jones infamy, when I was in medical school in India from the BBC radio[16]"

"It will be thirty years since the Jonestown massacre this year. I believe that the Guyanese government was so ashamed at having allowed him to build his state within a state that it tried to airbrush the massacre of innocents from history."

George "Jonestown happened way back in 1978 and things have changed enormously since then, Guyana is now a free democratic country and was even certified by the US Department of State as such"

"Do you need police escort when we are in Guyana?"

George "Don't be silly! It is probably safer in Georgetown than walking down Hillside Avenue or the streets around Brookdale University Hospital."

George is always ready with facts and figures "The year 2007 was regarded as one of the most successful for the police, when serious crimes declined from 16 per day to 9 per day, a 24 percent decrease. The murder rate for 2007 year was the lowest since 2002 with 113 for the year[17]."

George "I already took the liberty to find out that you are not on call on the weekend – March 2008, and you are coming with us to check out the story of the kid from Guyana who is dying and needs a kidney transplant."

George "The weekend we fly is Phagwa in Guyana, which is a Hindu festival of colors, it will be fun."

Phagwa or Holi (as it is called in much of the Indian diaspora and in India) is not much celebrated in the US, although it is becoming a little more popular with an increase in immigrants of Indian origin. Diwali[18]–the festival of lights and the Indian New Year is more popular even with the second and third generations of Indian immigrants.

I grew up in India, and Holi was always very popular, having left India in 1982, I never got the chance to celebrate Holi. Most of my visits back home to India were in the winter months of November and December when the heat and humidity are less oppressive.

16 http://news.bbc.co.uk/onthisday/hi/dates/stories/november/18/
    newsid_2540000/2540209.stm
17 http://www.gina.gov.gy/archive/daily/b080503.html
18 http://en.wikipedia.org/wiki/Diwali

The meaning of Phagwa is derived from an ancient Indian language – Bhojpuri, also called the "Festival of Colors". A large number of Guyanese trace their ancestry to the Indian province of Bihar in Northern India, where Bhojpuri is spoken. Phagwa is essentially a Hindu spring festival and is observed in India, Guyana, Trinidad, and Nepal. In West Bengal, it is known as Dolyatra or Boshonto Utsav ("Spring Festival")[19]. On the first day, Phagwa is celebrated by a ritual burning of the demoness Holika, Hiranyakashipu's sister in a huge bonfire at night. On the second day, known as Dhulheti, people spend the day throwing colored powder and water at each other. There is a theory that in the spring season, during which the weather changes, is believed to cause viral fever and cold. Thus, the playful throwing of the colored powders has a medicinal significance: the colors are traditionally made of Neem, Kumkum, Haldi, Bilva, and other medicinal herbs prescribed by Ayurvedic doctors. In some parts of India, a special drink called thandai is prepared, sometimes containing bhang (Cannabis sativa) to celebrate Phagwa; some of these rituals have become even more popular with the growing audience of Bollywood films. Rangapanchami occurs a few days later on a Panchami (fifth day of the full moon), marking the end of festivities involving colors.

So, the deal was done. We will fly to Georgetown, Guyana, to check out the story of the kid who cried for help! George, Jaskaran Persaud, Lakeram Persaud and I will spend a few thousand dollars to check out the story which George found on a flyer on Hillside Avenue, Queens, New York City. We will also partake in Phagwa celebrations and sample some Guyanese food, see the sights and sounds of Georgetown and of course visit the Georgetown Public Hospital Corporation (GHPC).

George is indeed a man of great persuasive powers.

---

19   http://en.wikipedia.org/wiki/Holi (Holi takes place over two days in the later part of February or March. As per the Hindu calendar, it falls on the Phalgun Purnima (or Pooranmashi, Full Moon), which was on March 22 in 2008. On the first day (22 March 2008 CE), symbolic burning of evil takes place, while the fun part of playing with colors takes place on the second day).

Chapter 3:

Exploratory Visit to Georgetown, Guyana

George, Jaskaran, Lakeram and I set out to Georgetown to investigate the story of a young man who is dying of kidney failure and his mother is desperate to send him to India for a kidney transplant. She herself is the potential kidney donor, but she does not even know if she can medically donate a kidney, she may well have diabetes, hypertension or many conditions which may preclude her from undergoing surgery. And of course, she has very little money to enable her son to get a kidney transplant.

All we know that she is a vendor of green vegetables at the local market and on many days, she does not even sell enough to recoup her bus fare to the market. She is also a single mother, her husband left her for the US when he could not cope with his son's illness. We have no knowledge of his whereabouts and Munesh has not heard from his dad for over four years.

We take the flight from the John F. Kennedy Airport to Georgetown. Caribbean Airways has a direct flight to Georgetown with a brief halt in Trinidad. We land early in the morning on March 22nd, 2008. We take a rundown taxi to Buddy's hotel. George is upset as we were expecting a limousine, which did not materialize. Jaskaran was supposed to make the arrangements—so Jaskaran is in the doghouse.

George is a big man, and he likes to travel first class in the plane and usually has a big SUV to take him around.

George "What a start to our mission, no limo to take us to the hotel."

George "We had to wait an hour in the line to clear the customs, Jaskaran, where is the official who was supposed to meet us at the airport?"

The start to our mission was not good.

We finally arrive at the hotel—a large Western style hotel with a nice pool. Again, there was a mix up and the reception did not have the rooms ready for us. George was really upset, having traveled the whole night, and then no one at the airport to greet us, and then travel forty-five minutes in a small rickety taxi was taking its toll. The girls at the reception, were so slow—typical of everything in Guyana, life takes its own course, why hurry? And then there is nowhere to go any way—so why hurry at all?

After two hours of waiting, we finally manage to get our rooms, large comfortable rooms with a view of the pool and the new cricket stadium, a pride and joy of the country. The stadium was a gift of the government of India to the people of Guyana. Sri Lanka and West Indies were playing a "test match" during the days we were in Guyana and George had arranged to get a VIP box for a day to watch the game of cricket. Cricket is a national pastime in Guyana, as is in India—where cricket is a religion. The stadium was built by the Government of Guyana with substantial financial assistance from the Government of India. Seating 15,000 people, Providence Stadium dwarfs other sports complexes in Guyana, and now hosts test cricket instead of Bourda (Bourda being the internationally famous one, where test matches were played till the new stadium opened its doors. Some cricket experts consider it to be the most majestic and beautiful ground in the world). The complex includes a shopping mall and luxury apartments. Buddy's Hotel is located next to the stadium, and has numerous luxury guest rooms[20].

Passion for cricket is all pervasive in India, when we were growing up in India, whenever India was playing a test match, the entire country would stop to hear the running commentary. If the game was played in a particular city in India, that day would be declared a holiday. Guyana

---

20 Providence Stadium is located on the east bank of the Demerara River a few kilometers south of the capital, Georgetown. Located along the East Bank Highway the stadium is a ten minute drive from Georgetown's city centre and a 30 minute drive from Cheddi Jagan International Airport. http://en.wikipedia.org/wiki/Providence_Stadium

is part of the West Indies Cricket Board[21] that has produced some of the greatest cricketers—the off-spinner, Lance Gibbs, and the three Berbician middle-order batsmen, Rohan Kanhai, Basil Butcher, and Joe Solomon. Their contribution was continued or extended by the advent, in the 1960s and early 1970s, of three other Bourda heroes, the left-handed batsman, Clive Lloyd, Roy Fredericks and Alvin Kallicharran. I remembered vividly watching Rohan Kanhai, Alvin Kallicharran, Clive Lloyd in India.

The most successful Guyanese batsman at Bourda in this era was Butcher, who scored seven hundreds there, two more than Solomon, Fredericks and Kanhai. His success, however, was surpassed by Garfield Sobers who was the most outstanding batting hero at Bourda between 1956 and 1975. In this period he scored seven hundreds there, two in inter-colonial games and five in Tests, including a century in both innings (125 and 109 not out) in a Test against Pakistan in 1958. Sobers has the record for the highest number of runs and centuries in Tests at Bourda (853 runs, average 94.77). In recent times Bourda's main heroes have been the two local stars, Carl Hooper and Shivnarine Chanderpaul; we would later run into his dad at Buddy's hotel. Hooper's renown is largely the result of several good all-round performances which have contributed immensely to Guyana's success. Particularly impressive were his feats in regional tournament in 2001 when he scored 954 runs, including four-hundreds and four-fifties, in twelf innings at an average of 95.40 runs an innings, took eleven catches and captured twenty-five wickets at 25.42 runs each.

Chanderpaul's acclaim has been due mainly to his productive batting, especially in Tests where he has scored several centuries. In 1998, for example, he scored 118 against England, the first Test hundred by a Guyanese at Bourda in twenty-five years. Chanderpaul's most memorable innings at Bourda, however, is probably his uncharacteristically aggressive hundred against Australia on the first day of the initial Test of a series in 2003. Made off only sixty-nine deliveries, it is the third fastest Test hundred ever in terms of balls faced[22].

21 The West Indies is a sporting confederation of over a dozen mainly English-speaking Caribbean countries and dependencies that formed the British West Indies. http://en.wikipedia.org/wiki/Cricket_in_the_West_Indies

22 http://www.embguyana.org.br/Cricket.htm

Guyana played host to international cricket matches as part of the 2007 Cricket World Cup. The new 15,000-seat Providence Stadium, also referred to as Guyana National Stadium, was built in time for the World Cup and was ready for the beginning of play on March 28. At the first international game of CWC 2007 at the stadium, Lasith Malinga of the Sri Lankan team performed a helmet trick or double hat-trick (four wickets in four consecutive deliveries)[23.] George and I often talked about the cricketing stalwarts of our younger days. I did not realize that we had so much in common!

Although, I am a recent immigrant from India and George an immigrant from Guyana to the US, we have a lot in common—Indian heritage, although separated by 169 years. The majority of Indo-Guyanese are the descendants of the Indentured labourers who were brought from (then) British India, to what was then called British Guiana to work in sugar cane plantations after the abolition of slavery in 1833. These indentured labourers were firstly brought by ocean travel aboard the vessels Hesperus and Withby. Most Indo-Guyanese are Hindus; substantial minorities are Muslims and Christians[24][25]

George is active within the Indo-Guyanese community in New York, sponsoring the parade through Liberty Avenue, in Queens on Guyana Independence Day. I asked George if he could trace his forefathers to that ship which brought Indians to Guyana.

George "Yes, we have traced our family roots right up to that ship; on May 5, 1838 on the ships, Whitby and Hesperus, 936 Indian indentured workers after a hazardous journey crossing from Calcutta to then British Guiana. The descendants of Indian laborers in Guyana now number over 400,000 in Guyana and an equal number residing in the United States, Canada, the United Kingdom and countries of the Caribbean region."

Later, we would go and visit George's ancestral home in Bel Air, which is in the modern section of Georgetown very close to the beaches and meet some of his relatives and walk to the local shops, where George is treated as a hero from the United States who has made it big. George always carries with him US$100 dollar bills which he gives to many who come to greet him.

---

23 http://en.wikipedia.org/wiki/Culture_of_Guyana
24 http://en.wikipedia.org/wiki/Indo-Guyanese
25 Indians in Guyana: A Concise History from Their Arrival to the Present by Basdeo Mangru, ISBN-10: 0967009308

I was still catching up on sleep, having a severe case of jet lag when I was urgently summoned to a poolside conference with Dr. Leslie Ramsammy, the Honorable Minister of Health in the Guyana Federal Government. Dr. Ramsammy heard through the grapevine that a group from New York was in town to investigate the story of a young man who was suffering from kidney failure. In a small country news travels fast. I was taken aback that the minister himself would come to talk to us informally at our hotel.

Before, walking down from my room, I quickly googled Dr. Leslie Ramsammy and learnt that he earned his PhD at St. John's University in Queens, New York. After receiving postdoctoral fellowships in neurochemistry and nephrology, he became a professor of medicine at the State University of New York at Stony Brook. Dr. Ramsammy returned to Guyana in 1994 and was chosen as the health minister seven years later. Most recently, Minister Ramsammy was elected President of the World Health Assembly. He grew up in an impoverished community in Guyana. Dr. Ramsammy says he was always driven by a sense of service to others. As a young man, he hoped to be a journalist but ended up studying microbiology in the USA. Enjoying and excelling in his studies, he returned to Guyana during a time of political transition where he says he got "caught up in the development". And there he has remained until now, serving in a wide range of public office positions culminating in the post of Minister of Health in 2001.

Minister Ramsammy is a man in a hurry. He is intense and has a directness to him, which endears him to some. But he also has a legion of enemies; however, he takes this in his stride. The Minister has all the statistics at the tips of his fingers. Second only to Haiti in terms of the lowest per capita income among Latin American and Caribbean countries, Guyana has long struggled to keep health care at the forefront of its national goals. In 1990, more than sixty children per 1,000 were dying before their first birthdays and nearly ninety before their fifth. Although Guyana's population is small, its battles with infectious disease are epic—only three years ago, more than 5 percent of the Guyana's citizens were infected with malaria and nearly 3 percent with HIV. Malaria, a common problem for the Latin American and Caribbean nations, has been reduced from nearly 40,000 cases in 2005 to fewer than 12,000 in 2007. Antiretroviral treatment of HIV & AIDS has increased substantially as a result of private-sector-funded health programs. Increased numbers of cancer screening tests, child vaccinations, and anti-malarial bed net distributed are accomplishments of a nation that the minister claims is taking full advantage of the global health funding afforded to it[26.]

Dr. Ramsammy believes that global health must be driven by Member States and that countries must be clear about what they want. "We are too conservative in our global health standards," he says in an interview. "A child born in Tanzania should have the same chance of survival and for living a healthy life as a child born in a developed country[27]."

He also cautions the health sector not to wait for perfect programs, techniques and interventions while people suffer. We must be practical and pragmatic about health interventions for communities, he emphasizes. That's why he came to meet us. Knowing well that Guyana does not have the infrastructure for a kidney transplant program and there were only four hemodialysis chairs for the entire country[28,] Minister Ramsammy was open to doing something about patients suffering from kidney failure.

Ramsammy "Most patients in kidney failure die or try to fund a transplant in India."

"Why India?"

Ramsammy "In India, it costs 10 percent of what it costs in the United States."

"What about the travel and family support?"

Ramsammy "The family has to go with the patient and they have to stay there for at least three months for follow up as most acute rejections occur within the first three months."

---

26 http://www.msh.org/news-bureau/health-minister-cites-positive-changes-in-guyanas-health-system-12-05-2008.cfm

27 http://www.who.int/mediacentre/events/2008/wha61/ramasammy/en/index.html

28 http://5gdialysis.com/about.html 5G, Guyana's first hemodialysis center, was established in order to satisfy the unmet need for dialysis in Guyana. Operational since July 2005, our dialysis centre is committed to providing for those in need of treatment and offers those who seek it abroad an affordable in-country alternative. We look forward to working with the Medical community and others to ensure that this treatment is available. The cost per treatment of long-term patients is US$175 and the cost per treatment of transient (visiting) is between US$200 and US$300.

"Of course, you can't send the patient alone without family."

"And who does the follow up, making changes in medications, monitoring for rejection, drug toxicity and potential surgical complications?"

Ramsammy "I don't know, patients perhaps return to India or communicate to the physicians in India by e-mails or telephone calls."

"Are there any local physicians who can follow up the transplant patients in Guyana?"

Ramsammy "I don't know. I assume some of the recently hired physicians from India may have had exposure to kidney transplantation."

"But, Guyanese traveling to India may become victims of fraud. In Toronto, a refugee who paid for a transplant in India ended up in Zaltzman's office with poor kidney function. Despite a six-inch scar on his abdomen, an ultrasound revealed there was no transplanted kidney and he was the victim of a con[29]." Probably more such cases of fraud may have gone unreported.

"Further, who is going to guarantee the quality of hospitals where the transplants take place? I know that donors have died in some hospitals in India, and there is no quality control outside of major hospitals[30]."

"Even more important is that the government of India has proposed a total ban on the donation of organs to foreigners by Indians, which may make it virtually impossible for Guyanese getting kidney transplants in legitimate hospitals in India[31]."

"What about doing kidney transplant here in Guyana?"

Ramsammy "Never thought of that angle, you think it is possible?"

"We shall have to see."

Ramsammy "Why don't you visit the hospital, meet with the local physicians and we will meet again in two days?"

---

29   http://www.commondreams.org/headlines01/0601-04.htm

30   Bansal RK. Donors do die in kidney transplantation in India. Indian J Med Sci [serial online] 2003 [cited 2008 Nov 17]; 57:320. Available from: http://www.indianjmedsci.org/text.asp?2003/57/7/320/11941

31   http://timesofindia.indiatimes.com/India/New_transplant_policy_to_curb_rackets/articleshow/3718196.cms

"We shall see if we can do the transplant surgery right here in Guyana."

The next few days were spent visiting Georgetown Public Hospital Corporation[32], meeting the physicians, laboratory staff, operating room personnel and ward nurses. We also visited some of the touristy places in Georgetown, which is on the right bank of the estuary of the Demerara River[33]. The site was originally chosen as a Fort to guard the early Dutch settlements of the Demerara River. The city lies below sea level and is protected from the Atlantic Ocean by the sea wall which was originally built in two phases. The first phase, up to the Roundhouse, was completed in 1860 and the second phase, extending to Kitty, was undertaken from 1872 to 1882. At the western end of the sea wall is a bandstand which was built in 1903. We walked along the sea wall from George's ancestral house in Bel Air up to Le Méridien Pegasus Hotel. This is a nice place to see the local people and perhaps chat to them informally. The wall serves a useful purpose as most of Guyana is under the sea level and it affords some protection from the high tides, however, floods still occur with depressive regularity bringing a number of infectious diseases with the water such as Leptospirosis and Dengue fever.

Georgetown is over two hundred years old. In 1781, the British military administrator of the recently captured colony of Demerara, Lieutenant Colonel Robert Kingston, established Fort St. George as his headquarters in a portion of the area presently known as Georgetown. The French gained control of the colony of Demerara in 1782. They demolished Fort St. George and built a new centre called Longchamps (La Nouvelle Ville). In 1784, the Dutch were once again in control of the colony of Demerara and they changed the name of their colonial capital from Longchamps to Stabroek[34].

We went up to the National Library, whose construction was funded by a Scottish-born American philanthropist Andrew Carnegie after whom the building was named. We also visited with President Bharrat Jagdeo, who is known to George. The State House is the official residence of the President of Guyana. The original structure was built in 1845 and it was known as Government House, the home of the Governors of British Guiana for over one-hundred years. The former

---

32   http://www.hiv.gov.gy/partner.php?id=3
33   http://www.geocities.com/thetropics/shores/9253/Rivers.html
34   http://www.guyanaguide.com/capital.html

Presidents of Guyana, Dr. Cheddi Jagan and his wife Janet Jagan lived in the building while Dr. Jagan was Premier of British Guiana from 1961 to 1964. The building is now the home of the Cheddi Jagan Research Centre which was officially opened on March 22, 2000[35].

On the way back after dinner at the Pegasus, we saw The Umana Yana and the Liberation, a short distance from Le Méridien Pegasus Hotel. The Umana Yana or meeting place of the people is a thatched benab built by the Wai Wai Indians for the Heads of the Non-Aligned Movement Conference in 1972. The Liberation Monument was unveiled in the forecourt of the Umana Yana during 1974. The monument commemorating solidarity with the African Liberation Movement and consists of five pillars of greenheart of irregular height and a slab of granite with pebbles around its base.

Other sites we saw were The Lighthouse, a brick and concrete structure about 31-metres tall, was built by the British in 1830 near the mouth of the Demerara River. It is the country's only lighthouse and guides ships into Port Georgetown with its revolving light. The National Park in Thomas Lands, formerly known as Queen Elizabeth Park, was opened by Queen Elizabeth II on February 5, 1966. Within the park are the Burrowes School of Art with a sculpture of Edward Burrowes on its roof, a sculpture in honour of scouting in Guyana and the Children's Millennium Monument.

The Indian Immigration Monument is located in a garden delimited by Camp, North, Alexander and Church Streets. The monument, a bronze replica of the vessel Whitby resting on a rectangular base, was unveiled on May 6, 1997 in commemoration of the arrival of the first East Indians in British Guiana. The vessel was one of two which brought the immigrants to the country on May 5, 1838. In the block bounded by Regent Street, New Garden Street and North Road is the Georgetown Cricket Club (GCC), commonly known as Bourda, where International Cricket matches are played. Cricket is one of the national sports of Guyana and Bourda is the only international cricket ground below sea level.

The Botanical Gardens on Vlissengen Road was originally laid out in 1879. It includes the Zoological Park, which was opened in 1952, parklands, flower gardens and a bandstand. A wide variety of birds, mammals and reptiles can be found in the Zoological Park.

---

35   http://www.jagan.org/

The roadways of the Botanical Gardens are lined with palm trees and manatees live in artificial lakes across which are bridges known as the Kissing Bridges. Recent additions to the Botanical Gardens are the Seven Ponds Monument (1969) and the Mausoleum (1986). Sir David Rose, the first Guyanese Governor General, and Martin Carter, a Guyanese poet are buried near the Seven Ponds Monument. The body of the First Executive President of Guyana, Forbes Burnham, is entombed in the Mausoleum. Sculptures by Ivor Thom, depicting the life and times of the late President, cover portions of the Mausoleum's interior walls.

At the corner of Vlissengen Road and Homestretch Avenue is the Castellani House, formally named in 1993 after its architect, Cesar Castellani. The original building was constructed during 1879 to 1882 and was the residence of the Government Botanist George Jenman beginning in 1883. Forbes Burnham resided there from 1965 until his death in 1985, during his tenure as Prime Minister and later, President of Guyana. The Castellani House is the home of the National Art Collection. The National Independence Monument, on Brickdam, near Vlissengen Road, is a gift to the people of Guyana from the Demerara Bauxite Company commemorating Guyana's Independence from Great Britain on May 26, 1966. The structure, in the form of an arch, consists of three tubes made of aluminum from Guyana's bauxite mounted on a quartz base. The arch was designed by a Canadian engineer, Edric Klak. A short distance east of the National Independence Monument, in the Square of the Revolution, is the 1763 Monument with a statue of Cuffy who led the 1763 slave rebellion at Plantation Magdalenenburg in Berbice. The bronze statue is the work of the sculptor Philip Moore. It is 5-metres high and rests on a concrete foundation designed by the architect Albert Rodrigues. At the corners of Mandela and Homestretch Avenues is the National Cultural Centre where theatre productions and concerts are held. It was opened in 1976. Poetry readings and plays were also staged by the Guyana Theatre Guild at the Kingston Playhouse[36].

Overall, Georgetown is an interesting city to visit with lots of historical places to visit within a few miles of each other.

---

36 http://wikimapia.org/1169101/Georgetown

Chapter 4:
Surprise Visit to the Mangal's Home

Although we had already spent two days in Georgetown meeting the Minister of Health, seeing the hospital, and visiting with the local physicians to gauge the possibility of carrying out the operation in Guyana, we still had to meet Munesh Mangal and his mother. In fact we had an appointment to see Munesh and his mother in the surgical ward of the hospital with their Nephrologist. So when we showed upon the ward at 10 AM, the appointed time, there was no one there to meet us. As we were leaving, George noticed a young man with his mother standing near the stairs to the ward. George likes to chat to people he meets here and there even if they don't know him.

George "What are you doing here in the sun, it's hot."
Munesh "Waiting for some doctors from the United States."
George "That's us!"

With that, George escorted Munesh and his mother to the ward.

Munesh is shy and hardly ever talks; he wears a towel over his shoulders to hide the dialysis catheter hanging from the right side of his chest. The catheter is used to access his blood stream for dialysis.

In the United States, we use a fistula or a graft connecting the artery and vein in the arm or forearm to puncture the fistula for dialysis[37]; clothing can hide this. However, in many countries where dialysis is just starting, physicians use a catheter as it gives easier access to the blood stream—cosmetically, it is not attractive, besides the fact that a catheter gets clogged up frequently and it has to be changed. We found that as patients could afford only short periods of hemodialysis and eventually died soon thereafter, there was no real indication for

37 Ryan JJ, Sajjid I, Jindal RM. ABC of vascular access for hemodialysis. Federal Practitioner 2005; 22:53-62.

placing a permanent vascular access for hemodialysis. In Guyana or other developing countries, the possibility of long-term dialysis does not exist as it is too expensive and patients simply die unless they can afford to obtain a kidney transplant.

We examined both the son and his mother thoroughly, and talked with them extensively to make sure they understood that a kidney transplant has never been done before in Guyana, and they would be kind of pioneers. Fortunately, the mother is extremely motivated and she understood the implications and potential complications of a surgery and its side-effects. Munesh understood the possibility of the transplant kidney not working, taking medications and life-long compliance with medications, and follow up care. He raised questions about the cost of medications, between US$8,000 and US$10,000, certainly prohibitive even for the well insured in the United States. We assured them that we would talk to the Department of Health about it.

We spent over two hours talking with them.

"What do you want to do after you get the transplant?"

Munesh "Go back to school and hang out with my friends."

"What do you want to do when you finish school?"

Munesh "Become the best car spray painter in the whole of Guyana."

"Why do you want to become a spray painter?"

At this point, the ward nurse overheard our conversation "His dad was a car spray painter and he left the family, so he wants to become a spray painter and show his dad how good he is."

Certainly, Munesh was determined to be the best car spray painter in Guyana, and why not?

At that point, our minds were made up.

However, there is always the nagging doubt that we may be made victims of fraud and they may not be really genuine cases of charity. So that evening, we drove twenty-five miles or so outside Georgetown to Lot 119 Lusignan Pasture, East Coast Demerara to see for ourselves how the Mangal family lived.

We went there unannounced and were taken aback by the poverty of the area and the condition of their house. The Mangal's have a single room with no inside bathroom. The shack is made of wood, and the only running water is from the tap outside which also serves as a bathroom. The front yard is full of junk, and materials from a car that his dad left behind. And there were also rusting cans of car paint in the front yard, a legacy of Munesh's dad who left them to seek his fortune in the United States. The family does not know of the whereabouts of Munesh's dad and he had made no attempt to contact the family for a couple of years. For all practical purposes, the dad may have been dead.

The Mangal's were surprised to see us; however, they were very gracious and showed us around their home—a single room.

The Mangal's house is in Lusignan; a village that is comprised of mainly indo-Guyanese and is sustained by subsistence farming. The community was brought to international attention following what has become known as the Lusignan Massacre[38]; a terrible event that left eleven persons, including five children, dead, after a group of heavily armed gunmen led by Rondell "Fineman" Rawlins stormed the village. All the eleven murders took place on the same street where the Mangals live. We visited one of the houses, four houses down from the Mangal's where both the husband and wife were killed. Rooplall Seecharan, fifty-six; his daughter, Raywattie Ramsingh, eleven; and his wife, Dhanrajie, called Sister, fifty-two, were killed in a hail of bullets[39]. We spoke at length to their son and daughter, who were still grieving at their loss. Guyana is still a country torn by inter-racial strife and violence—and we saw first-hand what it was by talking to some of the victims[40].

There was some Bollywood music in the background, evidence that some normalcy was gradually being restored in the drab lives of the people who live in Lusignan village and bravely face deranged gunmen who did not even spare children. I then learned that Bollywood is very popular amongst the Indo-Guyanese people. Bollywood is the informal term popularly used for the Mumbai-based Hindi-language film industry (Hindi cinema) in India[41.] The term is often incorrectly used to refer to the whole of Indian cinema; it is only a part of the Indian film industry. Bollywood is the largest film producer in India and one of the largest in the world. People of Indian origin, where ever they are, love Bollywood films and music. I listen to it when I

---

38 http://en.wikipedia.org/wiki/Lusignan,_Guyana
39 http://www.guyana.org/massacre_lusignan.html
40 http://news.bbc.co.uk/2/hi/americas/4270299.stm
41 http://en.wikipedia.org/wiki/Bollywood

drive to work and sometimes at home. I usually catch up on a couple of Bollywood films a month. I used to see a lot more of these when I was growing up in India, a time when the only entertainment was Bollywood. Bollywood films are mostly musicals, and are expected to contain catchy music in the form of song-and-dance numbers woven into the script. A film's success often depends on the quality of such musical numbers. Indeed, a film's music is often released before the movie itself and helps increase the audience[42].

We had tears in our eyes. George took out some US$100 dollar bills and gave it to them to make some basic repairs in the house. We wished the Mangal family well and told them that we are investigating the possibility of doing the kidney transplant right here in Guyana, however, we did not wish to raise their expectations too high.

On returning to the hotel, George insisted on having a dinner which included baigan choka, which is roasted eggplant, eaten on its own with Indian roti or nan bread or with chicken curry. It has intense flavor with wonderful texture. I love eggplant so when I saw this dish, I immediately ordered it with garlic and tomatoes. Originally, it was described as Trinidadian side dish or vegetarian spread for flatbreads, but is very popular with Guyanese around the world. Baigan choka tastes wonderful if eaten with roti; traditional Indian bread, made most often from wheat flour, cooked on a flat or slightly concave iron griddle. A good roti in Guyana is one that is very soft, with layers (almost like pastry layers if possible), which remains whole. The food in Guyana is certainly enjoyable with a mixture of Western, Chinese, Amerindian and Indian influences.

George likes baigan choka for breakfast as well as for lunch. He tells me that the recipe for this dish is well known, but not many people in the United States know about it. Essentially, the ingredients are eggplant, garlic cloves, tomato, onion, canola oil, scotch bonnet peppers, and salt. The eggplant is roasted until it gets soft, then it is slit and the pulp is scooped out and mixed with garlic, onion and pepper. It seems that the eggplant tastes better when roasted over an open flame. It is then cooked to taste and served with Indian breads.

We will carry out the groundbreaking momentous surgery in Guyana. Little did we realize that we will be under the microscope of the Guyanese press and the Ministry of Health till the surgery is complete.

---

42 www.bollywood.com

Chapter 5:

Social Network Analysis of the Guyanese Kidney Transplant

The kidney transplant required the coming together of four communities: Guyanese-American, Guyanese Ministry of Health, the United States transplant professionals and a team of Guyana-based doctors. The networks were linked by loose ties[43]. The networks that came together to help Munesh were evenly balanced in terms of power, skill base and support. The American-Guyanese business community had undertaken many goodwill health initiatives to their native Guyana in the past. Therefore, they were familiar with the socio-economic and political infrastructure of the country. The United States medical team, led by Dr. Jindal, had the medical skills to adapt to less sophisticated medical environments such as the operating facilities that they would encounter in Guyana. The medical team on the ground in Guyana, although lacking the skills needed to perform the transplant, were familiar with the patient's social networks and medical history. The Minister of Health and his team were ready to facilitate the teams and give an undertaking to provide free medications for at least three years (one year of anti-rejection medications costs about US$8,000).

Dr. Jindal and the United States medical team started to cultivate a working relationship via e-mail and telephone with the local Guyanese doctors as they worked up the patient. The flow of information between the medical teams supplied vital information for the sponsor (Mr. George Subraj) who was able to formulate their budget and manpower

---

43   The Struggle for life: A psychological perspective of kidney disease and transplantation, by LS Baines and RM Jindal. Publisher: Praeger, Westport, CT, USA, 2003. ISBN: 0-86569-323-4 (www.greenwood.com)

needs. It also provided George Subraj with positive reinforcement and motivation to pursue the mission.

The medical team in Guyana formed a professional network based upon a shared opportunity to fulfill a medical need within their country. The network was required to be highly flexible, in terms of making a number of timely transitions with regards to the role they played in the whole operation. In the early work up stages, they assumed a heightened role. However, once the United States-based team arrived in Guyana their role became both supportive by playing host to the visiting team helping them negotiate the logistics of hospital life. The Guyanese-based medical team was also privy to relational idiosyncrasies and external points of influence, such as the social networks in which the donor and recipient were embedded.

Dr. Jindal was clearly the 'star' or point of centrality that pulled together all four social networks. His centralized positioning meant that all information flowed through him and he was therefore in a position to influence the outcome of the transplant. Dr. Jindal used his position to ensure cohesiveness of the group and firm up inter-dependencies, minimize differences and prevent isolation between the four networks. He actualized this by ensuring that there were inter-connecting paths of communication between all four networks. This eliminated the potential for rigid boundaries and ensuring a balanced and harmonized network.

Dr. Jindal used his position of centrality to override any potential dysfunction.

Chapter 6:

Kidney Transplant Is Big News in Guyana

The news that Guyana will carry out its first kidney transplantation was covered in all the national newspapers. This put us under the microscope and intense pressure. Here are some of the news reports:

Lusignan Teen to Access Kidney Transplant at GPHC in July[44]

-To be conducted six times annually—
Ramsammy
By Melanie Allicock
A medical feat is expected to be performed at the Georgetown Public Hospital Corporation (GPHC) on July 12 when a 17-year-old boy from Lusignan on the East Coast of Demerara undergoes a kidney transplant. And, if all goes according to plan, the hospital will facilitate this surgery six times per year. The life-changing medical intervention will be led by two teams of more than 60 surgeons, nurses and other support staff from New York, and will be aided by local medical staff.

However the critical post-operative care will be carried out by local doctors. Describing it as a major step for the institution and the entire country, Health Minister Dr. Leslie Ramsammy said this latest move

---

44   http://www.guyanachronicle.com/ARCHIVES/archive%2012-07-08.
      html#Anchor--------------38541

will hopefully reduce the number of people having to travel abroad to take care of renal failure (kidney failure). This usually costs between US$15,000-$30,000 which is unaffordable to the majority of Guyanese. He noted that many kidney problems result from diabetes and patients in the past did not have an option locally once it was determined that dialysis could not work.

The US doctors will be volunteering their services as part of an arrangement with the Health Ministry to bring relief to the hundreds of Guyanese presently suffering from chronic renal failure. The cost of this initial venture will be not be borne by the patient or government, since a group of concerned US-based Guyanese have mobilized resources to cover the expenses that will be incurred by the medical team. He however disclosed government's plans of covering some of the expenses for future ventures of this kind.

He said that just like with the cardiac surgeries that began at the institution last year, the plan is to have local medical personnel undertake the transplant eventually.

"As time goes by the overseas team will get smaller and the plan is for the Guyanese doctors to eventually conduct the surgeries themselves, because part of the arrangement is for them to train our local doctors," the Minister noted.

Commenting on the 17-year-old patient, the Minister said he has been suffering from chronic renal failure for a while now and needs the transplant urgently.

Even though he was assisted by government with raising funds, he still could not access enough money to travel overseas to get the necessary medical intervention. His plight caught the attention of the team of doctors when they visited the country a few months ago. The boy's mother is the kidney donor for his transplant and, according to the Minister; the duo is ready for the critical surgery. All the tests have been completed and have revealed that the patient will benefit positively from the intervention "We have completed the angiogram and compatibility studies and we have confirmed that the patient and the donor are ready for the surgery," the Minister said The doctors, who will arrive in Guyana on July 9, will screen other patients with kidney disease.

A Stitch in Time
This intervention into the public health system could not have been timelier. Renal diseases contribute a major public health problem in Guyana, mainly because of the high incidences of diabetes and hypertension that exist. Guyana sees about 10,000 new hypertension and 8,000 new diabetes patients each year. These two conditions mainly result in kidney failure and account for a considerable portion of the more than 200 Guyanese in need of Dialysis treatment at the moment. As the prevalence of these two conditions continue to rise, more and more renal failure patients have surfaced, pleading for financial assistance through almost every medium available.

In the last year alone, this newspaper has highlighted the plights of more than 17 such patients. The sheer numbers of this phenomenon resulted in some fatigue on the private sector to provide ample financial assistance to these ailing Guyanese, making it more difficult for them to get support. Dr. Ramsammy said yesterday that one contributing factor to the high incidence of renal failure patients is the custom of waiting until very late before accessing care so that by the time the diagnosis for hypertension or diabetes is made, renal disease has already set in. He however noted that there are other causes for kidney disease including congestive heart failure, lupus, or sickle cell anaemia.

Guyana has struggled for a long time with dealing with the high incidence of kidney disease. Those who could afford to leave Guyana for dialysis treatment got temporary relief, but many of the less fortunate became very ill and died. In its bid to assist the situation, the Health Ministry offered a monetary assistance of US $5,000 to every patient, but for a person accessing dialysis care in Guyana at approximately US$200 per treatment, twice weekly, that money did not last long.

US-Based Help

Following the massive request for Guyanese to access transplants overseas, a group of Guyanese, comprising businessmen and other concerned citizens, mobilized themselves and began to solicit funds from overseas to help these patients. In the process, this group met doctors in the USA who decided that rather than only continue to donate money, it may prove more lucrative to provide of their services towards making a difference in the lives of these ailing patients. As such, a team of highly trained, experienced doctors from major hospitals in the US visited Guyana a few months ago to examine the health system.

Minister Ramsammy said these persons were pleasantly surprised at what they found.

"They came to Guyana with the perception that Guyana's health system was extremely weak and backward but they were pleasantly surprised that this was not the case and noted that with just a few adjustments, the GPHC could be made ready to facilitate kidney transplants without investing any money."

The Minister stressed that no infrastructural adjustments were necessary in order to prepare for the major operation, as the same theatre that was upgraded to facilitate the cardiac surgeries will be utilized. "In terms of equipment, no new ones were necessary, but the team needed a few pieces of surgical equipment." The angiogram machine at the Caribbean Heart Institute - used to examine the heart condition of patients - came in handy in the entire exercise since it is being used to examine the donor's kidneys to ensure their functionality. "We need to do that because to take out a healthy organ and leave an unhealthy one will accomplish nothing. "However, there are challenges in carrying out the organ compatibility studies needed prior to transplants.

An arrangement has been put in place for the doctors to conduct these tests at the hospitals in New York from which the doctors operate. In the initial stages, the Minister said only one transplant will be conducted at a time because of space limitations in the Intensive Care Unit of the GPHC, where the patients will receive post-operative care. "Because a kidney transplant is such a major operation, patients cannot be put in the regular wards. And remember that there will be two patients... the donor and the recipient...and we can't afford to occupy the ICU with just kidney transplant patients, especially in light of the upsurge of accidents in recent times."

Heart surgery patients are also placed in the ICU, for post-operative care, which puts an added strain on that ward. As such, the Minister acknowledged the need to expand the eight-bed ward in the near future. While government will not bear the cost for the actual surgeries-since the doctors will be volunteering their services - an exorbitant amount of money will be spent on post-operative care for which the hospital will have the responsibility. "The drugs that are needed are extremely expensive and while we already have some that are necessary in the system, the anti-rejection drugs that are critical are extremely expensive, and these are drugs that the patients have to take for months."

Dialysis Treatment in Guyana
The Dialysis program introduced in Guyana some years ago has brought some relief, but yet the vast majority of Guyanese in need of this service cannot afford it. A single dialysis treatment for patient with Chronic renal failure at Guyana's only haemodialysis centre, the 5G Dialysis Centre, costs in the vicinity of US$200 and in most cases is necessary twice weekly at the least. Some 200 persons are in need of dialysis treatment at the moment, of these 25-30 are accessing it outside of Guyana. Overall, less than half of these patients can afford to access the treatment. There are also a large number of overseas-based Guyanese with renal failure which have not returned home for years for fear of inadequate haemodialysis facilities. Minister Ramsammy said in acknowledgment of this, government has been looking at ways of making this service more affordable and announced yesterday that two additional dialysis centers will be opened within the next year. "Before the end of 2008 we will have the second dialysis centre open its doors in Guyana and if all goes well, a third by mid- 2009," he said.

The Central Islamic Organization of Guyana, in response to the crisis situation in Guyana had disclosed its intention of establishing a non-profit haemodialysis centre in Guyana before the end of this year. And Minister Ramsammy yesterday divulged that through a collaborative effort of Guyanese and overseas medical professionals, another such entity is poised to begin operations. The equipment to make this venture possible is already in the country, the Minister stated, adding that Guyanese will be able to benefit from the vast experience of these investors in the area of dialysis treatment at a reduced cost. "These groups are very experienced ... they actually operate existing dialysis centers in the USA, Canada, India and the Middle East ... because they operate others, the volumes of their purchases are garnered at significantly reduced prices so we expect that they will provide the services at a significantly reduced cost." He however stressed that dialysis treatment is not a cure but rather a "stop gap" and persons with chronic renal failure patients will eventually have to have a kidney transplant.

Kidney transplant negotiations took just over two months[45]

May 16, 2008 Source: Stabroek News

It took just over two months to wrap up negotiations so that the 17-year-old youth from Lusignan could get a much-needed kidney transplant which is set for July at the Georgetown Public Hospital.

Chief Executive Officer of GPHC, Michael Khan, yesterday said that he finalized the negotiations with Dr Rahul M. Jindal, who will be the lead doctor in the ground-breaking operation set for July 12.

It all began when Dr Jindal, a transplant surgeon at the Walter Reed Army Medical Centre in Washington, visited Guyana at the request of a Guyanese group which has been contributing to the health sector in Guyana for quite sometimes.

They heard about the young Lusignan boy who was a patient at the GPHC and was later told that he needed the kidney transplant. His family then launched an appeal to raise funds to get this done in

---

45   http://www.stabroeknews.com/news/kidney-transplant-negotiations-took-just-over-two-months/

India and through this appeal the Guyanese group heard of him.

After making contact with the boy, the group along with the doctor spoke with Minister of Health Dr Leslie Ramsammy.

Khan said at this point he became personally involved as the minister informed him that the doctor was interested in a tour of the hospital.

The doctor found the hospital's facilities to be suitable for such an operation and on his return to the US, he and Khan maintained regular contact via e-mail.

Khan said that at the hospital they are very excited and proud that such an operation could be done there following soon on the heels of the first open- heart surgery. It is expected that four kidney transplants would be done per year once all goes well, and all will be free of cost.

This would greatly assist local patients who have to find large sums of money to travel overseas to have the transplant done, often travelling as far as India.

Khan said at present they are checking to ensure that they have all the medications listed to be used after the surgery and if any is out of stock they would have it delivered on special order.

Last week Saturday the boy's mother, who is his donor, had an examination done to ensure that she can donate the organ to her son.

"It is a tremendous boost for the health sector and it is all part of the thrust of the government to deliver good health care," Khan said. Dr Jindal would be assisted by both local and overseas-based doctors during the operation.

A release from the Health Ministry on Tuesday said the procedure would likely reduce the trips abroad by local patients suffering from kidney failure.

Chapter 7:

Preparations Begin for the Kidney Transplant

After returning from Guyana, we set about the tasks of coordinating the "work-up" of Munesh and his mother for the transplant; getting the medical team ready, and getting their licenses and travel plans; as well as preparing the local team in terms of the Operating Room, anesthesia, Intensive Care Unit, laboratory facilities, and nursing staff.

Some of the tests such as tissue typing and cross-match were not done in Guyana; we obtained blood samples to perform the tests in the Immunology Laboratory of Walter Reed Army Medical Center, Washington, DC. The staff of both hospitals was very gracious in donating their time and expertise.

A total of 300 e-mails were exchanged and over one hundred telephonic calls were made by me, George Subraj and other players to Guyana to coordinate this effort.

Below are some of the e-mail exchanges that capture the saga of preparation and final departure for Georgetown, Guyana. I should add that there was some suspicion and apprehension amongst the staff in both places, but as you will see from the e-mails, this was gradually overcome and trust was build between the teams; the medical team from Walter Reed, George Subraj and his team; medical, nursing and laboratory staff at GHPC and the Minister of Health, Dr. Leslie Ramssamy and his officials. In short, a social network was established to ensure the smooth and successful completion of kidney transplant.

RE: Request for clarification

From: rahul jindal

Sent: Tue 3/25/08 7:15 PM

To: Michael Khan, CEO, GPHC, Georgetown, Guyana

Cc: Dr. Leslie Ramsammy, Minister of Health

Dear Michael

Thank you for your e-mail. Firstly, let me thank you for your graciousness during our visit to your hospital.

1. The tests I noted are for the mother.

2. The mother also needs a CT angiogram as we discussed. This it to determine if we take the right or left kidney (we avoid the kidney with multiple blood vessels). Instead of CT angio, MRA to visualize the blood vessels to the kidney will also suffice.

3. Both mother and son need a recent chest x-ray, liver enzymes, and a HIV test, Hep C and Hep B test.

4. Both the mother and son need a lymphocyte cross match and a repeat of blood group.

5. The son needs routine CBC and electrolytes.

Post-operatively, the immunosuppression will consist of Prograf, CellCept and prednisone. Please let us know if the local pharmacy stocks these medications.

I have already taken the first steps in forming a team of surgeons, nurses and intensivist for the surgery.

I look forward to hearing from you.

Regards,

Rahul M. Jindal, MD, PhD, MBA

Transplant Surgeon, WRAMC and Uniformed Services University

From: Michael H. Khan
To: rahul jindal
Subject: Request for clarification
Date: Tue, 25 Mar 2008 22:32:10 +0000
Dear Dr. Jindal,
Reference is made to your request for tests to be done. Kindly advise/clarify is the tests required are for the mother or the son or both.
Regards
Michael H. Khan
Chief Executive Officer
Georgetown Public Hospital Corporation

Re: Request for clarification
From: Leslie Ramsammy, Minister of Health
Sent: Sat 4/05/08 10:44 AM
To: rahul jindal
Dear Dr. Jindal,
We are having the test results put together. Mr. Khan will email you this afternoon. Please contact me is there is any problem for me to follow- up. The problem is we cannot deal with many persons over this. All the clinical arrangements will be with you. When too many persons are involved we will have confusion.
I was unable to contact you on your cell phone. You can contact me on my cell (592) 624-_ _ _ _ or office number (592) 226-_ _ _ _.
Best Regards,
Dr. Leslie Ramsammy
Minister of Health

RE: Request for clarification
From: Michael Khan, CEO, GPHC, Georgetown, Guyana
Sent: Sat 4/05/08 11:45 AM
To: rahul jindal
Cc: Dr. Leslie Ramsammy, Minister of Health

Dear Dr. Jindal,

Please accept my sincere apology for not responding to you sooner.

Please be informed that the CT angio and MRA are not done in Guyana. All of the other requested tests were done except the lymphocyte cross match. We are currently in contact with CAREC, Trinidad to have that test done.

Kindly note that on Monday 7 April 2008, the results of the tests that were done by the Georgetown Public Hospital Corporation will be mail out to you via DHL.

Regards

Michael H. Khan, CEO, GPHC, Georgetown, Guyana

RE: URGENT - From Dr. Jindal

From: rahul jindal

Sent: Thu 4/17/08 1:11 PM

To: Michael Khan, CEO, GPHC, Georgetown, Guyana

Cc: Dr. Leslie Ramsammy, Minister of Health

Bcc: George Subraj, lakeram

Mr. Khan:

I have still not got the DHL packet even after 10 days. From the DHL web site, it seems that the packet is held up in MIAMI due to incomplete paperwork. Please see what you can do.

The team is meeting this Sunday (George and others) to finalize the dates for surgery. We cannot proceed till the tests are taken care of urgently.

Thank you.

Rahul

Rahul M. Jindal, MD, PhD, MBA

Transplant Surgeon, WRAMC and Uniformed Services University

Update

From: Michael Khan, CEO, GPHC, Georgetown, Guyana
Sent: Fri 4/18/08 1:54 PM
To: rahul jindal
Cc: ministerofhealth
Dear Dr. Jindal,

The Georgetown Public Hospital Corporation does not have the capacity to offer HLA AB and DR testing hence arrangements are being made to have it done at CAREC Caribbean Epidemiology and Research Lab in Trinidad.

We were advised by CAREC that it has to be done by appointment and we are in the process of trying to secure an appointment.

Regards
Michael H. Khan, CEO, GPHC, Georgetown, Guyana

Update

From: rahul jindal
Sent: Fri 4/18/08 5:46 PM
To: Michael Khan, (CEO, GPHC, Georgetown, Guyana)
Cc: ministerofhealth
Bcc: lakeram; subraj
Dear Mr. Khan

I will send the tubes for blood and get the cross-match done in my hospital in the US. Can you please get the angiogram done ASAP. I also spoke to Dr. Wilson of the heart institute and he is happy to do the study.

Tentatively, we plan to bring the team and do the surgery in the last weekend of MAY.

I am therefore, requesting you to expedite all the processes.

Rahul M. Jindal, MD, PhD, MBA
Transplant Surgeon, WRAMC and Uniformed Services University

RE: Update
From: rahul jindal
Sent: Mon 4/21/08 12:53 PM
To: Michael Khan (CEO, GPHC, Georgetown, Guyana); George Subraj;
ministerofhealth
Dear Mr. Khan
1. I received the lab results and x-rays from DHL. The packet was held up in Miami for 10 days as they claimed that your office did not do the complete paperwork for customs.
2. Please let me know the complete address for sending the tubes.
3. I personally spoke to Dr. Wilson and Dr. Doobey who have agreed to do the angiogram.
Dr. Doobey will take care of the long-term postoperative care after my team returns to the USA.
The entire team met on Sunday and we will provisionally come to your hospital from 29th May to first week of June. We hope to do the surgery the 31st May.
I would also request that the various anti-rejection medications we described earlier will be available before the surgery.
In addition, can you let other renal failure patients know that they can consult with my team in various aspects of dialysis, renal failure and possible kidney transplant. This service will be provided completely free.
Regards,
Rahul
Rahul M. Jindal, MD, PhD, MBA
Transplant Surgeon, WRAMC and Uniformed Services University

Update
From: Michael Khan
Sent: Wed 4/23/08 2:27 PM
To: rahul jindal
Cc: ministerofhealth
Dear Dr. Jindal
Please be informed that the results for the Echocardiogram that was done on Ms. Mangal will be ready in two weeks time as advised by the Caribbean Heart Institute. Ms. Mangal had the echocardiogram done on April 18, 2008.
The result of the ECG was just received and is being faxed to you now.
Regards
Michael H. Khan, CEO, GPHC, Georgetown, Guyana

From: rahul jindal
To: ministerofhealth
CC: George Subraj, gphchosp; lakeram
Date: Tue, 22 Apr 2008 15:26:57 -0400
Subject: RE: —urgent
Padmini
Please confirm with the Minister that I will be bringing my team on the 29th May, surgery will be done on the 31st May.
Please let me know by the end of today as we need to book tickets and arrange for leave, etc.
Thanks
Rahul M. Jindal, MD, PhD, MBA
Transplant Surgeon, WRAMC and Uniformed Services University

Living Kidney Transplantation in Guyana

From: rahul jindal

Sent: Mon 4/28/08 10:19 AM

To: tsubraj

Cc: lakeram

Responses:

1. Patient's name: Munesh Mangal, age 18 years, address: 119, Lusignan Pasture, east Coast Demerara, Guyana. He is on hemodialysis via a right sided permacatheter by Dr. Doobey in Georgetown. His renal failure is due to hypertension. He is hepatitis C and B negative, HIV negative, Na 143.6, K 4.20, cl 107.6, Creatinine 5.3, uric acid 3.3, calcium 7.1, magnesium 1.0Hb 10, WBC 4.7. Chest x-ray is normal, EKG is normal. Blood group is B positive.

2. Mother's details: Leelkumarie Nirananjan Mangal: Age 41 years old, address is same as the son. She has no hypertension, diabetes or any other physical issues. Blood group is B positive, EKG is normal. She is a suitable donor for her son.

3. Dr. Leslie Ramsammy, the Minister of Health has supported this surgery and program. His e-mail is ministerofhealth@____.com. I have been in communication with him and his secretary. You can obtain confirmation directly with his office.

4. The following doctors from Walter Reed AMC have agreed to perform this surgery free of charge (Dr. RM Jindal, MD, Transplant Surgeon; Dr. Edward M. Falta, Transplant Surgeon; and Dr. Melanie Guerrero, Intensivist).

5. The following doctors in Guyana will be involved in assisting during the surgery and post-operative care (Dr. Michael Khan, CEO, Georgetown Public

Hospital; Dr. Doobey, Head of Internal Medicine; Dr. Wilson, Radiologist).

6. Mr. Michael Khan (Tel: 592-623-_ _ _ _) and the Minister of Health (Tel: 592-226-_ _ _ _) in Guyana have assured us of their cooperation and after care for both the patient and his mother (who is donating the kidney).

Thanks for your kind consideration.
Rahul M. Jindal, MD, PhD, MBA
Transplant Surgeon, WRAMC and Uniformed Services University

RE: visit—urgent

From:rahul jindal
Sent: Mon 4/28/08 1:22 PM
To: Michael Khan
Cc: ministerofhealthBcc: gsubraj
Dear Mr. Khan:
The tubes (including the pre-paid return and custom clearance papers) were sent to you by FEDEX on 4/28/2008 (air bill # 8657 0221 4128). We will perform the tissue typing and lymphocyte cross match in my laboratory.
Important: The tubes should NOT be placed in ice. Please use adequate bubble packing to protect the tubes from breaking.
Please let me know the exact date and time when the angiogram will be done so I can call Dr. Wilson when he is doing the angiogram procedure.
Thanks
Rahul M. Jindal, MD, PhD, MBA
Transplant Surgeon, WRAMC and Uniformed Services University

FW: Munesh Mangal
From: George Subraj
Sent: Fri 5/02/08 11:14 AM
To: rahul jindal
Sorry, I changed the dates from June to July

From: George Subraj
Sent: Friday, May 02, 2008 11:11 AM
To: rahul jindal
Subject: RE: Munesh Mangal
(I am planning to send this email to the Ministry of Health after receiving your input. Please add or delete as necessary).

Today at 9:00a.m, as promised, I tried to reach you by Conference call with Dr. Jindal, however, the phone rang out and then went busy for 15-20mins. As you are aware a team of five (5) is scheduled to come to perform the Kidney Transplant. I will continue try calling you or you may contact Dr. Jindal (202) 782-_ _ _ _ or George (email or by phone (646) 879-_ _ _ _.

On our visit there, we will like to see other people before and after the surgery. We are scheduled to be there from July 10, 2008 - July 14, 2008 upon receipt of your confirmation, we will make all arrangements with regards to the flight accommodations ad other expenses.

P.S. At this time, we are still waiting on the angiogram, which is proposed for May 10, 2008. As per Michael Khan, your office acknowledged receipt of the tubes for the transmission of the blood sample for testing in Washington.

As stated above you may contact me on my cell or email and / or Dr. Jindal directly.

Sincerely,
George Subraj
166-07 Hillside Avenue
Jamaica New York 11432
Tel: (718) ----3331 Fax: (718) ----5139
Gsubraj
Sent: Friday, May 02, 2008 8:19 AM
To: rahul jindal
Cc: gphchosp; gsubraj; lakeram
Subject: Re: Cross-match tubes
Dear Dr. Jindal,

Hope all is well with you. Thank you for this information. I will follow up with Mr. Khan's office to verify if they have received the package and I will also update Minister.

Take care.
Regards,
Padmini
Secretary to Dr. Ramsammy, Minister of Health, Government of Guyana

RE: Crossmatch tubes
From: rahul jindal
Sent: Wed 5/07/08 11:10 AM
To: Michael Khan; gsubraj; ministerofhealth; tsubraj
Dear Mr. Khan:

Can you let me know if the blood samples left your hospital.

Also, please let your local Anesthesiology Department know about the procedure, so they can prepare. Also, one of your local Surgeons is welcome to scrub with us so he/she can start gaining experience in kidney transplantation.

Thank you,

Rahul
Rahul M. Jindal, MD, PhD, MBA
Transplant Surgeon, WRAMC and Uniformed Services University

Re: Crossmatch tubes
From: Leslie Ramsammy Minister of Health
Sent: Wed 5/07/08 1:25 PM
To: rahul jindal
Dear Dr. Jindal

Hope all is well with you. Thank you very much for your email. Dr. Shamdeo Persaud, the Chief Medical Officer of the Ministry of Health has requested to have the Curriculum Vitae, copy of certificates and their current license of all the Doctors coming. This is to ensure that the doctors are registered with the Guyana Medical Council so that they can start working as soon as they come to Guyana.

Also, he has requested to have copies of you and your teams travel itineraries.

For further information, Please contact us.
Thank you and take care.
Best Regards,
Padmini
Secretary to Dr. Ramsammy, Minister of Health, Government of Guyana

(No Subject)
From: rahul jindal
Sent: Thu 5/08/08 11:48 AM
To: gsubraj
George:

One of the physicians who is a Critical Care MD, has a question about malpractice coverage:

Hello, Rahul

I do have questions regarding malpractice coverage, since Ed and I are doing this on our personal time and not covered by WR or the government. How do we protect ourselves and our personal assets for potential (although I understand unlikely) legal issues? I have heard of physicians doing humanitarian missions who have been sued by patients from other countries (with the help of U.S. attorneys) despite the noble cause of the project. Can your friend, the financial sponsor, have his attorneys draft up a contract signed by all involved?

Mel
M Guerrero, MD
LTC, Critical Care, WRAMC

RE: Visit
From: rahul jindal
Sent: Fri 5/09/08 8:02 AM
To: Michael Khan; gsubraj; ministerofhealth; tsubraj
Cc: edward.falta
Bcc: eric.elster
Mr. Michael Khan, CEO, Georgetown General Hospital
Dr. Leslie Ramsammy, Hon. Minister of Health
Mr George Subraj, President and CEO, Zara Realty, New York
Mr Lakeram Prasad, Chief Engineer, Estee Lauder, New York

Dear Mr. Khan:

The Ministers office has already received the CVs for the license and other formalities. As we move close to the date of surgery, we can start planning.

1. We will be leaving on the 9th July, and will do the surgery on the 12th July (Saturday).

2. We will visit the hospital on the 10th and 11th to finalize the arrangements.

3. Please admit both the mother and son on the 10th to the ward. Both patients will stay in the ICU for 3-4 days after surgery. The son will require barrier nursing for a week to prevent infections.

4. Please ask your Anesthesiology (2 MDs) to be in-charge and check the patients and give anesthesia. We want as many of your physicians involved for they can eventually take over and gain experience.

5. I have already asked Dr. Doobey (Renal) for post-operative and long-term care. Please feel free to involve other Nephrologists in the care so they can get experience as well.

6. We will need anti-rejection medications, which I was told are available in Guyana (Solumedrol, prednisone, CellCept and tacrolimus, bactrim, antibiotics, Valcyte, pepcid, fluconazole) in enough quantities. If you have substitute medications, please let me know.

7. We will be grateful if your Infectious Diseases physician examines the recipient (son - Munesh Mangal) if we need to give INH prophylaxis for TB. Munesh needs to have PPD done next week. His chest x-ray is normal.

8. Please have one of your Surgeons (preferably - Vascular Surgeon) to scrub with us so that they can start gaining experience and be available for post-operative issues.

9. Please ask 2-3 of your operating room nurses to be prepared to help us with the case.

10. We will do a 'dry run' for the case on the 11th July with your team of nurses and Anesthesiologists before the actual operation.

11. We have already seen and spoken to your laboratory physicians and Radiologists, who should also be involved with our team.

My team will consist of 2-3 Surgeons, Intensivist and a nurse. We will be happy to see other patients with renal issues and potential transplant patients for the future in a special clinic on the 10th and 11th July.

Please send me the report of the angiogram on the mother and the films by FEDEX. For the angiogram please ensure that we visualize the renal vessels clearly. The mother should be well hydrated and should get antibiotics prophylaxis before angiogram. I will speak with Dr. Wilson (your Radiologist) while he is doing the procedure on the 11th June

Thank you for your attention.
Rahul M. Jindal, MD, PhD, MBA
Transplant Surgeon, WRAMC and Uniformed Services University

RE: Angiogram
From: rahul jindal
Sent: Fri 5/16/08 1:17 PM
To: Michael Khan; edward.falta; gsubraj; lakeram; ministerofhealth; tsubraj
Mr. M Khan, CEO, Georgetown Public hospital
Dr. L Ramsammy, Hon Minister of Health

Dear Mr. Khan

I received the angiogram by DHL today, on the mother who is donating the kidney. The pictures are of excellent quality. There is a single artery for each kidney. All the tests are now complete on the mother.

Please request your Infectious Diseases specialist to examine the recipient (Munesh Mangal) to rule out TB or other infectious issues. As you know, the cross-match was negative.

I am indeed pleased with all your efforts to help this poor family.

Sincerely yours,
Rahul
Rahul M. Jindal, MD, PhD, MBA
Transplant Surgeon, WRAMC and Uniformed Services University

RE: Angiogram
From: Michael Khan
Sent: Sat 5/17/08 2:22 PM
To: rahul jindal
Cc: ministerofhealth; madan

Dear Dr. Jindal

Please be informed that I received a telephone call from the Honourable Minister of Health, Dr. Ramsammy advising me that there is a Dr. Nicholson, Nephrologist out of Barbados who claims that the patient (Mr. Munesh Mangal) is a patient of his and as such he should have been consulted.

I have since spoken with Dr. R. Doobay, Consultant, Internal Medicine, GPHC who has advised me that the patient is a GPHC patient who sought Dialysis treatment at a private institution in Guyana. He also stated that Dr. Nicholson apparently has some affiliation with that Dialysis Centre. The bottom line however is that the patient is a GPHC patient but I still thought that you should be updated.

Regards
Michael H. Khan, CEO, GPHC, Georgetown, Guyana

PS. Please note that any future emails relative to the clinical aspects of this case must be directed to the Director of Medical & Professional Services, Dr. Madan Rambaran whose email address is madan@___. com. The emails can be copied to me.

Medication list

From: rahul jindal
Sent: Fri 6/13/08 5:24 PM
To: Michael Khan; gsubraj; ministerofhealth

Dear Mr. Khan:

Here is the list:

Solumedrol (intra-venous): 1 gram on day 1, 500 mg on day 2, 250 mg on day 3, 125 mg on day 4, 100 mg on day 5.
prednisone (oral): start on day 6 at 80 mg and reduce by 10 mg a week to 20 mg a day.
CellCept (oral): 500 mg twice a day for life-long.
Tacrolimus (oral): 5 mg a day for life-long.
Bactrim: 1 tablet a day for 6 months.
Antibiotics: Please have Ancef and Cipro i.v. and po for 5 days.
Valcyte (oral): 450 mg a day for the first 3 months.
Pepcid or Zantac or equivalent (H2 blocker) [oral]: 1 tablet a day for first 6 months.
INH (oral): 300 mg a day oral for 6 months.
Fluconazole: 1 capsule a day for first 3 months.
Also, please have Ringers lactate, Normal Saline and 2 units if blood for Munesh Mangal.

Rahul
Rahul M. Jindal, MD, PhD, MBA

Transplant Surgeon, WRAMC and Uniformed Services University

RE: Medication list.
From: Michael Khan
Sent: Mon 6/16/08 2:18 PM
To: rahul jindal

Dear Dr. Jindal,

Please be informed that I will be away on vacation from June 19 until July 7, 2008. Nonetheless, I have checked with our Pharmacy Manager and wish to confirm that we have the following medications from your list available:

MEDICATIONS THAT ARE AVAILABLE

Prednisone (oral)—we only have prednisolone
Bactrim—available
Antibiotics (cipro i.v. and po)—available
Equivalent (H2 blocker) (ranitidine—available
INH (oral): 300 mg—available
Fluconazole—available
Ringers lactate, normal saline and 2 units of blood—available

ITEMS THAT ARE NOT AVAILABLE:

Solumedrol (intra-venous)
Cellcept (oral)
Tacrolimus
Valcyte
Antibiotics (Ancef)

Kindly advise if your team will be bringing those medications that are unavailable or if the Georgetown Public Hospital should procure same.

Regards

Michael H. Khan, CEO, GHPC, Georgetown, Guyana

RE: Medication list.
From: Michael Khan
Sent: Tue 6/17/08 3:48 PM
To: rahul jindal
Cc: madan

Dear Dr. Jindal,

Please be informed that arrangements are being made to procure those drugs from your list that we do not have in stock.

As I have indicated to you, I will be away on vacation leave effective June 19 to July 6, 2008 as such all future correspondence should be directed to Dr. Madan Rambaran. Dr. Rambaran will also be responsible for forwarding the names of Anesthesiologist, radiologist, Nephrologist, surgeon, pathologist, OR nurse, Ward nurse and laboratory technician as per your request so that you can send them your pre, intra-operative and post-operative protocols.

By copy of this email Dr. Rambaran is advised accordingly.

Michael Khan, CEO, GHPC, Georgetown, Guyana.

RE: Medication list
From: Michael Khan
Sent: Fri 6/20/08 3:33 PM
To: rahul jindal

Dear Dr. Jindal,

Our Pharmacy Manager is seeking your clarification regarding the Tacrolimus (Prograf) (oral).

Are you requesting that we get 0.5 and 1.0 mg capsules for the patient for at least 3 months and after that, the dosage will be increased to 5.0 mg/day dose life-long. We need this information to confirm the order.

Kindly advice as soon as possible.

Regards
Fiona McKoy
Administrative Assistant for Mr. Khan, CEO, GHPC, Georgetown, Guyana.

Dear Dr. Jindal,

I am advised that you will be performing a kidney transplant at Georgetown Public Hosp. Please let me know what I need to do.

Regards.
Madan Rambaran.
Interim CEO and Chief of Surgery, GHPC, Georgetown, Guyana.

RE: Blood samples - urgent
From: rahul jindal
Sent: Tue 7/01/08 8:51 AM
To: Leslie Ramsammy; gsubraj; tsubraj
Cc: madan

Dear Dr. Rambaran:

Please see the correspondence below for your action. Please update me on each of the items so the operation can proceed without obstacles.

Thank you,
Rahul M. Jindal, MD, PhD, MBA
Transplant Surgeon, Walter Reed AMC

Sent: Wed 7/02/08 7:45 AM
To: rahul jindal
Dear Dr. Jindal,

I am not sure who you saw and spoke to but we do not have 1. Infectious Disease Physician 2. Vascular surgeon 3. Radiologist by name of Wison.

In terms of local staff I will seek to organize a team constituted by Dr. Doobay, Physician, Dr. Purohit Urologist and 2 Anaesthesiologists.

Regards.

Madan, Interim CEO and Chief of Surgery, GHPC, Georgetown, Guyana.

Final Crossmatch
From: rahul jindal
Sent: Fri 7/04/08 9:12 AM
To: arthur.womble; edfalta; georgetown_hospital@hotmail.com; gsubraj; Khan, Michael; ministerofhealth; tsubraj
The Hon. Minister of Health
Government of Guyana

Dear Dr. Ramsammy:

The final cross-match between the mother and son is negative (both are compatible). This clears the way for the transplant to occur as planned.

My special thanks to Ms Padmini Narain and hospital staff who have worked so hard to "work-up" the donor and recipient and taking care of the logistics of our mission. We look forward to working with your team and meeting with you next week.

Kind regards,

Rahul M. Jindal, MD, PhD, MBA
Transplant Surgeon, WRAMC and Uniformed
Services University

Kidney Transplant Surgery

From: georgetown hospital (georgetown_
hospital@_____.com)
Sent: Fri 7/04/08 5:40 PM
To: rahul jindal

Dear Dr. Jindal,

My sincerest apologies for not replying to your mails
sooner, I would however like to provide you with
the names and email addresses of persons from our
hospital who will be directly involved in the surgery.

1. Dr. Ravi Purohit (Surgeon)
2. Dr. Ramsundar Doobay (Consultant, Internal
Medicine)
3. Dr. Anita Florendo (Registrar, Internal Medicine)
4. Dr. Vivienne Amata (Anaesthesiologist)
5. Dr. Pheona Mohamed-Rambaran (Laboratory
Director)
6. Mr. Delon France (Medical Technologist)

Additionally, I would appreciate if you can confirm
whether you will be bringing along the necessary
instruments for the surgery or if these have to be
provided by the hospital, in which case a list would
be very helpful. Our pharmacy made every effort in
procuring the necessary drugs but had some difficulty
in acquiring a few and we are kindly asking your
assistance in bringing the following drugs along with
you:

1. Solumedrol 500 mg
2. Thymoglobulin
3. Campath
4. Daclizimab or Basiliximab

The above named persons are expecting to hear from you as it relates to pre, intra and post operative care of the patients. Looking forward to seeing and working along with you on your upcoming visit.

Melissa Rockliffe
Administrative Assistant for Dr. M. Rambaran, Interim CEO and Chief of Surgery, GHPC, Georgetown, Guyana.

RE: Kidney Transplant Surgery
From: rahul jindal
Sent: Sat 7/05/08 10:24 AM
To: georgetown hospital
Cc: anita_cumbermack; vtamata; pheonar;
Bcc: gsubraj; Khan, Michael; lakeram; ministerofhealth; tsubraj
📎 3 attachment(s)

Anesthesi...doc (27.0 KB), Renal Tra...doc (18.4 KB), kidney tr...ppt (399.8 KB)

If you're having problems downloading attachments, please sign in again and select "Remember me on this computer."

I enclose the various protocols we use, as attachment to this e-mail.

1. The anesthesia protocol is attached. We will have our own anesthetist (Dr. Arthur Womble) who is very experienced however; Dr. Amata should become familiar with the protocols as she will be involved with pre-and intra-operative case. Also, Dr. Melanie Guererro will be coming with us. She is a certified Criticial Care and Pulmonary specialist.

2. I enclose an excellent evidence-based learning site for kidney transplantation from the American College of Physicians:

(http://pier.acponline.org/physicians/procedures/ physpro700/indications/physpro700-s2.html).

I am the current editor of this module. Please use my password to access this (pierguest; pier 12). It gives evidence-based information on all aspects of kidney transplantation, patient information, medications, complication and literature. All the information on this site is current and is updated by me every 15 days.

3. For this particular case (Munesh Mangal), we will be using Solumedrol induction, so we will not require Thymoglubulin, Campath or Daclizimab or Basiliximab, as there is a good match between the mother and son. We may require the other antibodies in future cases.

4. We will bring Solumedrol with us.

5. We will bring vascular clamps and sutures with us. However, we will require a standard general surgery tray of instruments for each case. You already have this as it was shown to me when I visited your hospital.

6. I also enclose a power point which I use to give a lecture to residents on kidney transplantation. It is an overview on the subject. It should be used in conjunction with the American College of Physicians module - Pier web site).

7. Finally, both the mother and son should be admitted 2 days prior to surgery. The patient (Munesh Mangal) should have full dialysis on the day of admission and on the day of surgery). He should have CBC and full chemistry on admission and day of surgery.

If you have other patients who may require kidney transplant in the future, please have detailed medical records ready for our review.

Sincerely,
Rahul M. Jindal, MD, PhD, MBA
Transplant Surgeon, WRAMC and Uniformed Services University

Anesthesia
From: Vivienne Mitchell
Sent: Sun 7/06/08 6:49 AM
To: rahul jindal
Dr. Jindal,

Thank you for your email. Could you please give me Dr. Wombles email address? I am simply the acting Head of Department, with effect from today. Dr. Harvey, the Head, is on her way to New York to undergo a Fellowship in cardiac Anesthesia.

The two Anesthetists here will be Dr. Andrew Amata who worked with patients for renal transplant at OHSU, Portland, Oregon and Dr. Yu Li from China, who also has experience with renal transplant anesthesia.

We lack many very basic items which Dr. Womble would reasonably assume we have. I have submitted a list to Dr. Rambarran, the Medical Director and continue to await a response from him.

Sincerely
Dr. Vivienne Amata
Chief of Anesthesia Services, GPHC

RE: Anaesthesia
From: rahul jindal
Sent: Mon 7/07/08 12:09 PM
To: Vivienne Mitchell
Cc: georgetown_hospital@_____.com; gsubraj; Khan, Michael

Dr. Amata:

We will try to get these.

We can do without CVP line. The drop method of counting will work for now as syringe pumps are bulky and will require custom clearance.

We could have got all the items if we had the

Sincerely,
Rahul M. Jindal, MD, PhD, MBA
Transplant Surgeon, WRAMC and Uniformed Services University

List from Georgetown
From: rahul jindal
Sent: Mon 7/07/08 12:14 PM
To: gsubraj
Tony:

We need to get these. I just got an e-mail from them.

1. Oro-pharyngeal airways.
2. Heat and Moisture Exchange filters (HMEF).
3. Isoflurane.
4. 0.5% bupivacaine for epidural analgesia.

Thanks,
Rahul M. Jindal, MD, PhD, MBA
Transplant Surgeon, WRAMC and Uniformed Services University

Re: missing items for anesthesia
From: Womble, Arthur L LTC RES USAR USARC
Sent: Mon 7/07/08 1:58 PM
To: rahul jindal

Dr. Jindal,

I was thinking about your question as to if we need these items. The airways may be needed but only 2 or 3. I will bring some. HMEF's are a great idea if they do not have them. We would only need 3 or 4 and are widely available. Florane is hard to get as I explained. Most institutions (ours included) do not utilize it anymore and do not store it. Army FSTs do still carry it though. I can get boat loads of bupivicaine.

Arthur Womble
CRNA, PhD
LTC, AN, USAR

RE: missing items for anesthesia
From: rahul jindal
Sent: Mon 7/07/08 2:34 PM
To: Womble, Arthur L LTC RES USAR USARC

Arthur:

I agree, besides I just realized that these are explosive and will not be allowed on the plane.

Rahul M. Jindal, MD, PhD, MBA
Transplant Surgeon, WRAMC and Uniformed Services University

RE: missing items for anesthesia
From: rahul jindal
Sent: Mon 7/07/08 7:41 PM
To: vtamata; georgetown_hospital; gsubraj; Khan, Michael; ministerofhealth; tsubraj

Dr. Amata:

I understand, not your fault. I have been trying to get Dr. Rambaran name the team at your end for over a month. As you know, the team and work at our end was complete a while ago. Dr. Womble will get the missing items, however, we cannot get liquids in the plane.

Anyway, we will do the 2 cases under GA, as there is better control, CVP is not essential, as long as the patients are in the ICU for a few days after surgery.

Hopefully, all will go well. All this work and effort is for the benefit of an extremely poor family and a young kid. As you know, none of us are taking any money, all this effort is entirely voluntary. The effort is being supported by Mr George Subraj and your Department of Health.

We hope that in the future, many more patients in Guyana will benefit from kidney transplants and will not have to travel to India or the USA at great cost and will benefit the medical community in Guyana. I hope my team and your physicians will work together in a spirit of collaboration and altruism.

Sincerely yours,

Rahul
Rahul M. Jindal, MD, PhD, MBA
Transplant Surgeon, WRAMC and Uniformed Services University

Chapter 8:
Kidney Transplant Successful

The press release from the Ministry of Health summarizes the first kidney transplant, I have re-produced it verbatim:

Sunday, July 13, 2008
Landmark kidney transplant operation a resounding success

The first local kidney transplant was successfully completed ahead of the scheduled time yesterday, thanks to the hard work and dedication of the medical team which undertook the task. The surgery to transplant a kidney from 41-year-old Leelkumarie Nirananjan Managal of Lusignan, East Coast Demerara, to her son, 18-year-old Munesh Mangal began at 7.30 am and was completed just after 2 pm.

Lead Transplant Surgeon at Walter Reed Army Medical Center in DC and Attending General Surgeon at the Brookdale University Hospital, Indian-born Dr. Rahul Jindal, said that the surgery was without complication and that both the recipient and donor are awake and recovering at the Intensive Care Unit, at the Georgetown Public Hospital (GPHC). He made this disclosure at a press conference yesterday at GPHC after successfully completing the operation. He explained that the mother is expected to remain at the ICU for another day, after which she will be transferred to the ward and then discharged. While her son will remain at ICU for about three days and once he is stable, will be sent to the ward for monitoring for another week.

"His kidney is making urine. We don't expect any problems later on," Dr. Jindal said, but noted that there is always the possibility that the lad's body might reject the new kidney. He however, noted that adequate medication would be provided to minimize the possibility of rejection and the next 48 hours remain a critical period for the recipient.

"It is a difficult operation. You only have one chance because if you fail and the kidney is dead, others are not easily available," stated Dr. Jindal.

According to Dr. Jindal the patients will have to remain on medications for the rest of their lives. He emphasized that while surgeries are helpful, prevention is better and urged all to take heed of preventative measures, some of which include regular exercise and proper diets and positive lifestyles.

"We are hoping that it will not be looked upon as just a transplantation surgery, but the beginning of the preventative measures of such kidney failures," said Dr. Jindal.

Minister of Health, Dr. Leslie Ramsammy welcomed the success and noted its another milestone for the Georgetown Hospital and Guyana.

"This is a truly historic day in our country it is a celebration of partnership and a milestone for the Georgetown Hospital and the country. We celebrate the local and international professionals who came together to truly achieve what is a miracle. This means so much to the health sector and to our country. We have worked successful to complete the first kidney transplant in our country," asserted the minister.

Dr. Jindal expressed gratitude for the confidence placed in him by local authorities and the family to do the surgery and noted that his involvement was prompted when he learnt of the family's financial difficulties in providing treatment and care for the sick child.

Munesh suffered renal failure years ago because of hypertension. He has been ill for most of his childhood, but in 1995 he began experiencing chest pains and was suffering from shortness of breath.

His condition took a turn for the worse last year, preventing him from attending classes at the Apex Academy, where he was preparing to sit the Caribbean Secondary Schools Examination, but never had the chance to do so. Munesh was diagnosed with End Stage Renal Failure last October while a patient at GPHCs clinic and it was then that the mother decided to undergo preliminary tests to determine her chances as a possible donor to her son. After numerous tests, she was confirmed a positive match and the overseas doctors agreed to do the surgery here. This was much relief since this surgery would have cost US$100,000 in the United States.

In March this year, Dr. Jindal was introduced to the local health sector and arrangements were put in place. Kidney transplant is a surgical procedure involving heterotopic placement of the donor kidney into the iliac fossa of the recipient. It has emerged as the preferred means of renal replacement therapy for patients with End-Stage Renal Disease of any etiology.

The leader of the medical team stated that the surgery created confidence in the local institution and has also created expectations and hope for other renal failure patients. On this note he announced that Government will be sustaining the effort to ensure that other patients benefit from similar options.

George Subraj, one of the sponsors of the initiative committed to procuring sponsorship for another five transplant surgeries and the health minister noted that the idea is to ultimately have local capacity to perform kidney transplant.

Dr. Ramsammy said at present there are about 200 Guyanese who should be on dialysis for renal failure and a portion of them would require transplant. Meanwhile, the Chief Executive Officer of GPHC, Mr. Michael Khan expressed his appreciation with the overseas team in performing the surgery free of cost and is looking forward to future collaboration with the group. He said the exercise will benefit the local doctors tremendously and it is hoped that very soon they will be able to perform such surgeries with little or no outside assistance.

The team will be staging a clinic at GPHC for other patients with similar conditions during their stay in Guyana. The team includes businessman George Subraj and his son, Tony; Lakeram Persaud, Jas Persaud and Kewan Totaram, as well as Caribbean Airlines, which sponsored the tickets for the visiting persons. And, according to Mr Subraj, yesterday's undertaking could be regarded as the beginning of an ongoing programme of assistance, even as he estimated that he would probably be able to bring the team back a few more times to conduct about five more operations. The medial team has already examined about six patients, two of whom may be eligible for surgery, according to Dr. Jindal.

The minister pointed out, though, that while the undertaking was one of success, there will still remain challenges for a mother and a child who will need prayers and understanding. He, however, assured that the health sector has in fact gained much, and by extension the country has gained. He also commended Dr. Jindal for finding the courage to even consider taking on the operation. But, according to the minister, it sometimes takes more than just professionals to complete a good job, thus other kinds of assistance were required.

In addition to the undertaking being a partnership of expertise, the minister said that yesterdays operation also shows how the Diaspora can help in development. "The Diaspora has been an important component in Guyana's development for over a decade now. Many of our programmes are tied to this contribution…"

In the end, we have succeeded in another milestone in our country, with a great bit of dignity and integrity of the process in place, and with two people having the chance at better lives and a promise in our country of a better health sector. Assisting Dr. Jindal from the overseas medical team were Dr. Edward M. Falta (Transplant Surgeon of the Walter Reed Army Medical Centre (WRAMC), Washington), Dr. Melenie Guerero, (Pulmonary Care Physician), Laura Owens (Transplant Coordinator) and Dr. Arthur L. Womble attached to the Athens-Limestone Hospital, Athens, Alabama. They arrived in Guyana last Thursday. The local team includes Dr. Ravi Purohit (Surgeon), Dr. Ramsundar Doobay (Consultant, Internal Medicine), Dr. Anita Florendo (Registrar, Internal Medicine), Dr. Vivienne Amata (Anaesthesiologist), Dr. Pheona Mohamed-Rambaran (Laboratory Director), Mr. Delon France (Medical Technologist) and Dr. Wilson (Radiologist).

Source: The Guyana Chronicle[46]

---

46   http://www.guyanachronicle.com/ARCHIVES/archive%2013-07-08.html

July 15, 2008
Team awarded for successful kidney transplant

... Momentous occasion in Guyana— Ramkarran

After conducting a successful kidney transplant for the first time here in Guyana, the team of doctors which made the operation a success was last evening presented with awards, indicating Munesh Mangal's (the kidney patient) appreciation for giving him another chance to live.

Caribbean Airlines, Buddy's International Hotel and the Neal and Massy Group were also awarded for their participation in making the surgery a successful one. All told, those who received awards were Dr. Melanie Guerrero, Dr. Edward Falta, Dr. Arthur Womble, Dr. Rahul Jindal, Nurse Laura Owen, Jas Persaud, General Manager for Caribbean Airlines, Carlton Defour, Mr. Sanders also of Caribbean Airlines, Neal and Massy representative, Shameer Hoosein, and Om Prakash Shivraj.

Special mention was also given to Tony Yassin, Health Minister Dr. Leslie Ramsammy, and Publisher of Kaieteur News, Glenn Lall among others for their contribution toward making the surgery a success. The initiative to have the operation done in Guyana was spearheaded by New York-based Guyanese, Mr. George Subraj, after he saw a flyer that was being circulated for financial assistance for the kidney patient. The awards ceremony, which was held last evening at Buddy's International Hotel in Providence, East Bank Demerara, attracted Chief Executive Officer of the Georgetown Public Hospital Corporation, Michael Khan and Speaker of the National Assembly, Ralph Ramkarran. Mr. Ramkarran noted that the success of the kidney transplant is a momentous occasion for Guyana and he thanked the surgeon, Dr. Rahul

Jindal, for giving life to Munesh Mangal. "When I heard about the project two months ago, I became immediately sympathetic. I understand the trauma of finding money every week for dialysis treatment," Mr Ramkarran said. In a case like this, the doctors and the supporting team dedicated their willingness, time, energy and resources to make it a success, Mr Ramkarran said. The man who put together the entire project, George Subraj, said the venture was not an easy one, as there were a lot of stumbling blocks. He, however, noted that more such transplants will be conducted here in Guyana, as he committed to facilitate at least five more kidney transplants.

Subraj explained that when he first heard of Munesh Mangal's problem he started to investigate. When he came to Guyana and visited the family's home in Lusignan, East Coast Demerara, Subraj said that tears came to his eyes, as he realized how poor the family was. Dr. Rahul Jindal who conducted the surgery said that it is a unique story for Guyana. He explained that the 18-year-old is recovering favorably at the hospital, and he is in 'high spirits'. Mr. Subraj, who facilitated the entire process, sought the assistance of Caribbean Airlines which sponsored the tickets for the team; the owner of Buddy's International Hotel who accommodated the team at a reduced rate; and a few others who have helped in the area of providing meals for the team since their arrival here in Guyana.

Meanwhile, Mr. Subraj has not only assisted Guyana medically, but has also helped in the Information Technology field. Recently, he facilitated the construction of a computer laboratory at the Cove and John Ashram. It was revealed last evening that another such laboratory will be constructed there some time this year. By Knews[47]

47 http://www.kaieteurnewsonline.com/2008/07/15/team-awarded-for-successful-kidney-transplant/

Minister of Health

MINISTRY OF HEALTH - Lot 1 Brickdam, Georgetown, Guyana, South America.
Tel: 592 226 1560 Fax: 592 225 4505 E-mail: ministerofhealth@gmail.com

July 31, 2008

Dr. Rahul Jindal, MD, PhD, MBA
Transplant Surgeon, Walter Reed AMC
6900 Georgia Avenue NW
Washington, DC 20307

Dear Dr. Jindal,

Re: The First Kidney Transplant in Guyana

On behalf of the Ministry of Health and the Georgetown Public Hospital, I extend warm congratulations to you and your team for the successful completion of the first kidney transplant surgery in Guyana. More importantly, we would like to express our profound gratitude to you and the team: Dr. Edward M. Falta, Dr. Melenie Guerero, Ms. Laura Owens and Dr. Arthur L. Womble.

The surgery added to the morale of the staff of the GPHC and in many ways has contributed to the upgrading of the services in general at the GPHC.

We appreciate the professionalism of the team and the graciousness with which the team conducted their work.

Let me also on behalf of the Mangal family (Mrs. Mangal and Munesh) express their gratitude.

We look forward to a continued engagement with the team and hope that this service will develop as a permanent programme at the GPHC.

Again, our deepest gratitude to you and the team.

Sincerely,

MINISTRY OF HEALTH
JUL 2 1 2008

Dr. Leslie Ramsammy, MP
Minister of Health, Guyana

71

Thursday, August 21, 2008
Walter Reed Doctors Perform Guyana's First Kidney Transplant [48]

By Sharon Taylor Conway

Stripe Staff Writer

Lt. Col. Edward Falta, chief of the Walter Reed organ transplant service and Dr. Rahul Jindal, Assistant Chief, performed the first kidney transplant operation in the Co-operative Republic of Guyana, July 12.

The landmark, living donor surgery involved two simultaneous operations: harvesting a healthy, compatible kidney from a 41-year-old mother for transplant to her 18-year-old son in end stage renal failure. The teenager's kidney function was so poor that Jindal said the situation was like throwing the dice every week on how long he would survive.

Jindal led the team of five Army medical professionals who traveled to the small, South American country, the size of Idaho, for the humanitarian effort. The group trained their Guyanese medical counterparts.

Falta and Jindal, along with Lt. Col. Melanie Guerrero, a Walter Reed Army Medical Center critical care physician, Spc. Laura Owen, a WRAMC transplant technologist, and Art Womble, a certified nurse anesthetist from Athens-Limestone Hospital in Athens, Ala., who donated their skills and vacation time to perform the milestone surgery. The Walter Reed team members perform about 30 transplants a year at WRAMC.

Falta explained all the critical pre-operative lab tests were conducted at Walter Reed, such as tissue-typing,

---

48 http://www.dcmilitary.com/stories/082108/stripe_28214.shtml

cross-match. Walter Reed has the only HLA (human leukocyte antigen) lab in the military and one of the oldest in the country, according to Falta. The team used WRAMC surgical instruments and returned them to the hospital after the operations.

It took four months to set up the infrastructure necessary to perform the procedure at Georgetown Public Hospital. From their WRAMC location, the Walter Reed team supervised operating room preparations and staffing.

It all began when the teenager was diagnosed with kidney failure two years ago. Soon after, he quit school, suffering chest pain, general malaise and chronic fatigue. He received dialysis whenever his single mother, who worked as a roadside vegetable vendor, was able to scrape the money together.

Sometimes the bus ride into town to sell the vegetables cost more than what she was able to make Jindal said.

According to 2006 United Nations statistical data, the per capita annual income in Guyana was $1,219 compared $43,562 in the United States.

Dialysis is a very expensive life-saving procedure and in Guyana it costs $500 cash per session. And, we usually require three times a week and these people have to pay out of their pockets, so for a developing country it was a big problem. A huge economic drain on the community, on the government and the people themselves, Falta said.

The struggling mother tried every way she could to raise money for dialysis. When a flyer soliciting funds landed in the hands of a Guyanese philanthropist living in Queens, N. Y., the wheels were set in motion for the ground-breaking surgery.

Jindal explained original efforts were geared to find money to send the teenager to India for a transplant. They do surgery at the cost of one tenth that in the United States. It costs $150,000 for a transplant here. In India, it ís $35,000. But Dr. Leslie Ramsammy, Guyana minister of health and president of the World Health Assembly had another idea.

Ramsammy suggested that the surgery be done, in country. It would be a big boost there were 250 patients [needing kidney transplants], and they can't afford to send all the patients to India, Jindal said.

A kidney transplant is still cheaper than dialysis, Falta said. Here in the United States, dialysis is shown to decrease your lifespan five to eight years.

Jindal was open to the idea, pondering whether they could teach transplant techniques to the Guyanese surgeons and step back after a few years, leaving them to perform the procedure on their own.

When he [Jindal] came and described the situation it was the exact same thing I tried to do on my own, Falta said.

In 2004, Falta attempted to save 16-year-old Honduran girl in renal failure, waiting six months to navigate the U.S. government administrative and logistical channels. The girl died from inadequate dialysis before Falta could receive the green light to perform the transplant.

Guyana's first kidney transplant operation took nearly seven hours to complete, without complications. Jindal said the transplant recipient's prognosis looks excellent.

Through phone calls and e-mail, Jindal helps the medical staff in Guyana manage the follow-up health care management issues that arise. The Guyanese government will pay for the medicine the teen must take for the rest of his life.

A full month after the epic surgery, the young patient is doing well. He is back in school, enrolled in Information Technology classes.

The surgery added to the morale of the staff of the GPHC [Georgetown Public Hospital in Guyana] and in many ways has contributed to the upgrading of the services in general at the GPHC, Ramsammy said.

Transplantation makes a good humanitarian instrument for the U.S. government because it is long-term and turns a negative situation into a positive one. [The patient] doesn't just stop dialysis but he goes back to school and back to work ó he contributes to society instead of being a drain, Falta said.

Jindal's next transplant mission trip to Guyana is scheduled for Nov. 12, when he plans to do two more kidney transplants. The government of Guyana has promised to supply post- transplant medications free to the first 20 patients.

On November 3, 2008
Kidney transplant patient now leads a more active lifestyle[49]

By Iana Seales

- Caring for sick mother
Munesh Mangal has a candid tongue, so when he speaks it is interesting to listen, and after three months of recuperating from his kidney transplant surgery, he has quite a lot to say, particularly about how his days

---

49 http://www.stabroeknews.com/news/kidney-transplant-patient-now-leads-a-more-active-lifestyle/#comments

are no longer humdrum and filled with the agony of knowing he was dying.

The 11 years he had suffered with defective kidneys now resemble a bad horror story he was once caught up in and he insists on putting them behind him. His immediate focus is on staying healthy, keeping out of hospital and resuming classes, which he was forced to quit a few years ago.

Since his groundbreaking surgery on local soil in July, he had been hospitalized for a period of two weeks — the stent that had been placed inside him had to be removed and re-inserted.

On the day of this interview, Munesh was found sitting at the medical clinic at the Georgetown Public Hospital after a regular check-up with the doctor — he is required to visit twice a week – looking at a piece of paper that holds the results to a blood test he had taken the day before. He is deep in concentration, almost unaware of the presence of his sister nearby and the countless other persons waiting to see the doctor. After a long, hard study of the results he looks up and says that the doctor was right; he is okay.

Munesh then runs off to the pharmacy, returns with his medication and sits down. He is ready to open up. His medication is a combination of drugs that he is required to take twice a day. In total, he swallows 10 pills in 24 hours. But he says that if 100 pills a day would keep him healthy then he would happily ingest them all.

"I am not too bothered by the regular routine of drinking pill after pill twice a day what does worry me is that they keep changing. One time I had certain strength then another time I received another so I was a bit confused and I asked the doctors about it. Now things are okay I think," he says.

Doctors say that Munesh's medication is also being monitored as he responds to it so it is likely that he could be on different pills, different weeks but they are aiming for uniformity.

The 19-year-old says he has good days and others when he feels like his body has taken a severe beating. In the early days of his post-surgery recuperation, he was constantly plagued with aches about the body, and had no choice but to lie in bed and sleep the pain away. But that was in the past since he is hardly ever at home these days.

Call it a burning desire to be on the road again, but Munesh has been hanging out and reconnecting with old friends within the past month. There was a time when he knew what was on television at specific hours; now he has trouble remembering time slots. He sees the change as a progressive step towards his long-term recovery since being active is a prerequisite.

Munesh is somewhat troubled that his mother, Leelkumarie Mangal, has not been able to adapt to a more active lifestyle since surgery. Since she gave him one of her kidneys he believes it is only fair that she gets use to walking around some more and "getting off the bed that she is so attached to."

Munesh is close to his mother, so close that he often sits down and decides what is best for them both, and most times she finds it agreeable. They live alone at their Lusignan home and had been doing so for a few years now. His parents are separated and he has an older sister who has married and moved out. If his mother falls ill, he somehow finds the strength to press on without her, as he was forced to do at the time of the interview.

Leelkumarie is hospitalized and had been for four days before he sat down with Stabroek News. Her condition is not listed as serious but doctors are closely monitoring her; the incision she received during surgery is developing an abscess. She had not been hospitalized prior but there were moments of severe pain.

Munesh recounts it as though he personally suffered, but again he points out that she has not been as active as prescribed. Stabroek News also spoke with Leelkumarie, who struggled to sit up in her hospital bed, and refused to lie down when encouraged to do so. She, too, is frank, spilling that from the outset her road to recovery has been rough. It is nothing doctors had not previously said to her, but still, it is more than she had imagined. However, she underscores that giving up one of her kidneys for Munesh is the sacrifice that any healthy mother would make.

"Sometimes I do feel like I am always going to have to battle something or the other since the surgery but seeing him walking around looking so healthy I am just happy and thankful," she says, staring at her son as she spoke.

There was so specific medication prescribed for her after surgery; doctors simply told her to take better care of herself. Leelkumarie said she has done nothing but follow their advice, yet her condition continues to raise questions as to whether she should be on medication.

Questioned about this, Minister of Health Dr. Leslie Ramsammy said she is being monitored regularly and that doctors have been positive about her recovery. He said the doctors would only prescribe medication as required, noting that Leelkumarie has been on a few pills but not more than is necessary. Both mother and son are under the care of Dr. Purohit at the public hospital, the minister said, adding that they are receiving quality care.

Leelkumarie does not dispute what the minister said, but says she hopes her condition improves and that someone can take a closer look at her current medication and see if any changes should be made. She is also hoping that the pain would ease; constant pain that has plagued her since the surgery.

Munesh is at the hospital regularly; he takes her meals, which he prepares himself and hangs around until visiting hours end. Twice a day he is at her bedside and if he had it his way, he would be there all day keeping her company. He speaks to her with deep concern in his voice, asking whether she had breakfast and if she is in need of anything in particular. As she lies on the bed responding to his battery of questions, the roles are reversed—he is like the parent fully in control, for now.

Indo-Guyanese George Subraj Honored[50]

On Sunday, July 20, 2008 in Queens, New York, members of the Indo-Caribbean Counicl (IIC-NY) and Shri Devi Mandir welcomed Shri George Subraj, a PIO born in Guyana, to bestow upon him The Councils highest honor. Giving meaning and expression to its mission to "recognize Indo-Caribbean's and to serve others," The Council invited Shri George Subraj to receive this accolade for his financial, moral and humanitarian support of the first kidney transplant in Guyana, which was performed at the Georgetown Hospital. In fact, this is the first kidney transplant in the English-speaking Caribbean. Reflecting its plural composition, Council members Shri R.D. Kalicharran, Dr. Tara Singh, Hajee Zakir, Rev. Seopaul Singh, Shri Lalbachan Haricharran and

---

50 http://www.gopio.net/news_081508.htm

Shri Roopnarain Persaud were in attendance at the temple to receive and welcome the honoree, Shri George Subraj.

Not only did Shri George Subraj contributed financially to the successful operation, he personally involved himself in all the logistics, permits and clearances from Government Ministries and hospital personnel. One could have expected complete cooperation from Guyanese officials; this however was not the reality. It was an uphill struggle to secure the necessary "paper works", and, if Shri George Subraj did not personally involve himself in securing the permits, the operation would not have even occurred, much less become the success it has been recorded to be. George Subraj's philanthropy deserves, and is here given, its rightful place in the history and maturity of the Indo-Caribbean group of People of Indian Origin.

The eight-hour operation was conducted by a U.S.-based medical team headed by Indian-born Dr. Rahul M Jindal of Brookdale University Hospital. Other members included: Dr Edward Falta, Transplant Surgeon of the Walter Reed Army Medical Centre (WRAMC), Washington; Dr. Melenie Guerero, Pulmonary Care Physician; Laura Owens, Transplant Coordinator; and Dr. Arthur L. Womble, attached to the Athens-Limestone Hospital, Athens, Alabama. The local team comprised: Dr. Ravi Purohit, Surgeon; Dr. Ramsundar Doobay, Consultant, Internal Medicine; Dr. Anita Florendo, Registrar, Internal Medicine; Dr. Vivienne Amata, Anaesthesiologist; Dr. Pheona Mohamed-Rambaran, Laboratory Director; Delon France, Medical Technologist; and Dr. Wilson, Radiologist.

Munesh Mangal is recovering well, and so is his mother, who donated one of her kidneys to him. They were discharged from hospital on Monday, July 21, 2008. Munesh is responding well to treatment and George and Lake returned to Guyana on Tuesday, July 22, 2008, to monitor and help provide post-operative care to the Munesh Mangal's family. The Guyana government has promised to supply at least three years medication to Munesh. "If this is done right, then we will be on the right track to carry out similar transplant cases in the future." observed Shri George Subraj in his acceptance remarks. He continued in his remarks to give thanks to each and everyone who assisted in fulfilling the need of the sick.

PART II

Chapter 9:
Munesh Becomes Non-Compliant

Why do patients become non-compliant after receiving a life saving organ? Do some patients have a 'death wish'[51]? Munesh was doing very well, when at 9 weeks after receiving a kidney transplant, he stopped taking his medications. This happened when he was well enough to start Information Technology classes. George Subraj had arranged and paid for a one-year course of Information Technology hoping that he will acquire skills which are sought both in Guyana and other countries and be able to support himself and his mother.

The onset of non-compliance is interesting. When Munesh presented to the hospital with a rising serum creatinine suggesting various possibilities: rejection of the transplant; mechanical obstruction of the ureter carrying urine to the bladder from the transplant; toxicity from prograf (one of the anti-rejection medications) or perhaps dehydration. Patients on dialysis are advised to restrict their fluid intake, so it can be difficult to increase the fluid intake as is mandated for a recipient of kidney transplant. The physicians at GPHC had to work with one hand tied behind their back as they did not have facility for taking a kidney biopsy (although the biopsy could technically be done, there was no Pathologist to read it) and Prograf toxicity could not be ruled out as GPHC did not have the laboratory equipment to perform drug levels. It is very expensive to set up a drug assay system for just 1 patient.

Dr. Purohit admitted Munesh to the hospital for tests gave him <u>empirically</u> intra-venous fluids to correct dehydration and after a lot of

51 Jindal RM, Joseph JT, Morris MC, Santella RN, Baines LS
     Noncompliance after kidney transplantation: A systematic review.
     Transplant Proc 2003; 35:2868-2872.

telephonic discussion with me over the phone from Guyana, decided to place a "ureteric stent" to correct possible urinary obstruction. Trying to find a pediatric ureteric stent was another issue. I was in India visiting my family, when I got a call from Dr. Ravi Purohit describing the situation and he was at his wits end as the hospital did not have a pediatric stent, biopsy facilities or techniques to determine drug levels. Having come so far, working under the glare of the media, made us nervous, but more determined.

I called Tony Subraj and George Subraj from Ahmedabad in India (I always have my cell phone on even when I am travelling for conference or social visits). George was in Toronto, Canada, making a deal as only he knows how! However, he is always approachable and he picked up the phone (it was 3 AM in India). We arranged for the ureteric stent and anti-rejection medications to be flown to Georgetown, Guyana.

After 24 hours of giving Munesh intra-venous fluids, his creatinine came down slightly from 4.3 to 4, but 4 is still too high and suggestive of severe kidney dysfunction. After more calls back and forth, Ravi Purohit decided to take Munesh to the operating room and place a ureteric stent which he happened to find in the operating room of GPHC. Ravi himself went looking through hundreds of boxes of materials that have been left by various charitable organizations that visit Guyana. Placing a ureteric stent in a transplanted kidney is more difficult than placing a stent in a native ureter. However, using his vast experience, Ravi was able to successfully place a ureteric stent.

At first, Munesh denied being non-compliant; as you will see from the discussion later on, this is common – denial. However, when Ravi confronted him, he agreed that he was indeed non-compliant. After a long discussion, it was still not clear why he became non-compliant. Perhaps, we were not sufficiently clear about the timing and dosage of medications or the inevitable side effects of medications. Perhaps we were not empathetic and Munesh did not trust us. To put it bluntly, we told him that the eyes of the whole of Guyana are on him–a good result will enable more Guyanese to get transplanted. A bad outcome would be the end of the program. Well, I then received this from Ravi:

From: ravi
To: rahul jindal
Subject: Re: Munesh—urgent
Date: Fri, 19 Sep 2008 00:48:35-0400
Rahul,

NON COMPLIANCE. Today I scrutinized them
again & though they denied it initially, Munesh later
accepted that he was irregular with his medicines.
Past few days, since he started going to school, he
was not feeling well after taking Prograf & Cellcept
& so has taken only half doses of each. I explained
& warned him. Hope he will be compliant in future.
Tony called me today & gave his number [I was in
the operation room]. I spoke to him later & also
mailed him necessary information. The stent I have
used is 16 cm [appears about 2 cm extra in length]
but I think should not bother him much. Tomorrow
I will remove the Foley catheter. Today evening we
have sent sample for Cr estimation I will let you know
once results are received.

Ravi.

Munesh responded to steroid pulse and placement of the stent.
Usually, we treat one condition, presumed rejection, but in view of the
lack of biopsy facilities, lack of drug levels, we decided to go ahead and
place both the ureteric stent and treat him for acute rejection.

Re: Munesh - urgent
From: Ravi Purohit
Sent: Sat 9/20/08 7:46 AM
To: rahul jindal
Rahul,

His latest Cr is 3.0, I did not inform you yesterday
because there was some confusion about the timings
when the samples were drawn [before or after the last
dose of solumedrol]. It is still not certain but we decided

to repeat it in next visit. Clinically, he is showing elevated BP [intermittently in 140/90 range? effect of steroids/saline hydration] Dr. Doobey suggested 2.5 mg nifedepine. He was very keen on going home & at that time I thought it was a risk [with so much of steroid immunosupression] to send him home with indwelling catheter & removed it If you strongly feel it is necessary I will call him & re-introduce it. He will be coming for check up on Monday/Tuesday. I will let you know the fresh lab results then.

Ravi

Gradually, Munesh responds to treatment:

Date: Wed, 29 Oct 2008 17:59:47 -0700
From: pinkryhan
Subject: Re: Munesh
To: rahul jindal

Dr. Jindal, I am sorry about responding so late, we had a few problems with the laboratory at GPHC, blood had to be sent out:

Labs:
Bun-31mg/dl
creat-2.1mg/dl
Ca-7.8mg/dl (8.5-11)
Mg-1.3meq/L (1.3-2.5)
P-2.8mg/dl (2.8-5.0)
Meds:
Cellcept 1g bd
Prograf 1mg bd
Valcyclovir 450mg on alternate day
Septrin 960mg on alternate day
prednisolone 15mg po od
Amlodipine 2.5mg po od
Omeprazole 40mg po od
Dr. Singh, Medical Officer, Department of Medicine, GHPC, Georgetown, Guyana

WHY DID MUNESH BECOME NON-COMPLIANT?

An esoteric explanation for Munesh becoming non-compliant is whether he was forgetful or trying to make a point or showing his independent from the rigors of dialysis by "taking his life in his own hands—a show of bravado?" Our line of thinking is based upon the belief that all patients contemplate non-compliance, but for the majority of the time comply with the treatment regime. Overtly, these patients are very critical of their fellow non-compliant patients. However, during therapy, compliant patients will often relate to a specific non-compliant patient with great compassion, concern for their wellbeing and relief that someone was not so accepting of our predicament. It is as though compliant patients can maintain their position, safe in the knowledge that someone else is articulating their own frustration, fear and anxiety so they do not have to do so. In brief, they are mindful that their feelings are being represented, albeit by proxy.

TREATING MUNESH'S NON-COMPLIANCE

Relentless striving for incremental improvement can make progress. This can be achieved in designing better and improved cars, saving money or losing weight. We believe this principle of incremental improvement can be applied to increase in medical compliance with medications and the transplant process itself. The treatment of non-compliance in this setting has been fragmented and non-uniform. Ultimately, the transplant community needs an inclusive model capable of detecting and treating the non-compliance before it proves fatal. In our own transplant unit, we have being working towards such a multi-faceted approach using psychotherapeutic principles as a means to detect, understand and treat non-compliance amongst dialysis and transplant patients. This work is based upon our understanding of the patient's experience of renal disease and organ transplantation as recalled during psychotherapy.

WHAT IS NON-COMPLIANCE?

We have discussed various forms of non-compliance extensively in my PhD thesis[52] and also in our book[53]. Compliance amongst patients undergoing dialysis and after transplantation has become an important issue as non-compliance with the primary treatment regime leads to complications and even death. The problem of non-compliance is thought to be particularly acute amongst the lower socio-economic groups (Bame et al. 1993, Leggat 1998), in patients between 20-30 years of age, females (Leggat 1998) and in black patients (Alexander 1998). Furthermore, patients who do not adequately comply with dialysis are less likely to be placed on the waiting list for kidney transplants. This is particularly true in women from black or lower socio-economic groups who are more likely not to complete the transplant selection process, and therefore, have higher rates of morbidity than those patients who do comply and receive a kidney transplant (Alexander 1998). It has also been shown that patients identified as non-compliant with dialysis who did receive a kidney transplant were more likely to lose their graft or die after transplant (Alexander 1998).

However, despite the pivotal importance of compliance behavior amongst this patient group, a concise definition and standardized measurement of the concept remains illusive and effective intervention is not well defined. This situation is worrying as considerable attention has been given to measuring and predicting compliance, despite there being no consensus between various centers as to what is being measured and predicted.

Traditionally, compliance behavior has been considered in terms of the physician's ability to influence the patient and the patient's willingness to respond. However, in an attempt to move away from connotations of the all powerful physician and the powerless patient, there was a move to replace the term 'compliance' with that of 'adherence' and more recently with 'concordance'. 'Adherence' and 'concordance' play to the contemporary espousal of a more empowered patient and

---

52 Jindal RM. PhD thesis (2004). Middlesex University, London, United Kingdom. Improving quality of life, emotional states and medical compliance in recipients of kidney transplants.

53 The struggle for life: A psychological perspective of kidney disease and transplantation, by LS Baines and RM Jindal. Publisher: Praeger, Westport, CT, USA, 2003. ISBN: 0-86569-323-4.

a more egalitarian physician. However, legislation that translates into real world empowering of patients has been lacking and may be the primary reason that the term 'compliance' has prevailed and therefore will be referred to as such throughout the book.

Patients who do not comply with the medical regimen and lose their grafts may be denied a second transplant, an area of considerable controversy and debate. Furthermore, health care financing is assuming a central role in our society. Patients who lose their transplants due to non-compliance will result in significant drain on finances as these patients are placed back on dialysis, a modality of treatment more expensive than a functioning transplant. Medical non-compliance is also important as it is estimated that over 25 percent of patients who enter into clinical trials of anti-rejection drugs may be non-compliant and hence influence the results of these studies.

A number of authors have studied various factors that affect medical compliance after kidney transplantation. These include demographics, social and educational status, mental and behavioral patterns, pre- and post-transplant symptoms and beliefs, and the characteristics of the transplanted recipient. A variety of validated instruments have been described to assess and in some cases predict non-compliance after a kidney transplant. These methods include pill counts, clinic attendance, drug levels and self-administered questionnaires. Each of these methods has pitfalls and may not be equally applicable to all patients.

Indeed, it would seem that transplant patients tend to be divided into those who comply with the treatment regime and those who do not. Non-compliance with dialysis is not necessarily an accurate predictor of post-transplant compliance and should not always be used as a means to exclude patients from the transplant program. However, patients with a history of non-compliance with dialysis are liable to feelings of fear of a recurrence of non-compliance behavior which might jeopardize their transplant, but over which they feel they have no control. They may have symptoms of anxiety, insomnia and guilt at having received a kidney from a cadaver source and hesitancy regarding the future, accompanied in some cases by low mood. These mood states can be effectively treated using short-term psychotherapy aimed at increased understanding of past non-compliant behavior. In turn, such insight creates a more stable and productive mood state and facilitates actualization of a better quality of life in the future (Auer 1982). Skotzko et al. (2001) carried out a survey to determine the views of the transplant community on psychosocial issues. They found that there was overwhelming support for providing psychosocial support both pre- and post-transplant to increase compliance and rehabilitation of patients. There was also a broad support for substance abuse treatment programs for recipients of organ transplants; most respondents also acknowledged the impact of psychosocial factors on compliance, quality of life and survival. Respondents to this survey also pointed to the need for formal studies of psychosocial intervention on cost and resource utilization, which will convince health service planners to adequately fund such programs. We agree with these authors that standard practice guidelines need to be formulated for psychosocial intervention, in particular, for training of health care providers working with recipients of organ transplants.

GENETIC BASIS FOR NON-COMPLIANCE?

Burnham and Phelan in their book 'Mean Genes' have proposed that our actions and lives are governed by a set of 'mean genes', against which we are engaged in a constant battle. The temptation is to follow the path of least resistance and simply live our lives as our urges and passions direct. The alternative path is the path of most resistance. Medical non-compliance can perhaps be considered in this context. The path of least resistance, which is not to take medications, however, the same genes have also given us the power of self-control. These authors suggest that in addition to the genes that get us into trouble, we have genes for free will and self-discipline. Therefore, it is also within our genes to find the tools to fight our animalist urges and take control of our lives.

Furthermore, new genes are being discovered for aging, alcoholism and other aspects of human behavior. Genetic influences have clearly more influence on human behavior than previously assumed and it is also becoming apparent that our evolutionary inheritance plays a central role in our lives. Is there a gene for 'medical non-compliance', or indeed for 'compliance'? We know there are pleasure centers and putative genes for addiction in the brain, so it is not such a far-fetched idea, as it first seems. Given the central role of dopamine in pleasure centers in the brain, it may even be related to compliance or risk taking behaviors leading to non-compliance. This is an intriguing question we will have to consider in later years. It is clear that seemingly normal, motivated persons deliberately decide to become non-compliance with their anti-rejection medications and go on to lose their transplants and eventually die. Do these persons carry a 'death wish'? It is indeed puzzling why people derive pleasure from taking risks. As suggested by Burnham and Phelan, we should start looking at human behavior by understanding Charles Darwin and not Sigmund Freud.

MEASUREMENT OF NON-COMPLIANCE AMONGST PATIENTS RECEIVING DIALYSIS

The techniques of measuring non-compliance have, in the main, been analyzed in terms of apparently tangible constructs. These include a single or combination of measures at either one point in time or over a specified period as follows:

Transport records and interviews: Non-compliance measured in terms of shortening and researchers at the Vanderbilt Dialysis Clinic, Nashville, USA investigated missing dialysis visits. They used a series of interviews and transport records, which they related to doses of hemodialysis received (as determined by hospital records), to assess whether or not this group of patients was compliant. They found that a significant number of shortened treatments were due to delays in hospital transportation, but missing treatment visits were thought to be related to other undefined variables. The authors used their findings to stress the need for ongoing educational programs to encourage compliance (Latham 1998).

Fluid volume excess: Fluid volume excess has frequently been used as a means to measure non-compliance with hemodialysis. Fluid volume excess is measured by weight gain, peripheral edema, and abnormal pulmonary findings taken before each hemodialysis treatment. Subsequent measurements were used as a means to determine ineffective management by patients of their hemodialysis treatment (Sciarini 1996). This technique remains one of the commonest measures of non-compliance in patients receiving hemodialysis.

Biochemical data: Investigators measured the mid-month blood urea nitrogen, serum potassium, and phosphate values of 54 maintenance hemodialysis patients at regular intervals over the course of a six month period to determine compliance with hemodialysis (Arici et al. 1998). Their analysis revealed deviation in compliance of a significant number of patients. The authors suggested that the monitoring of biochemical indicators was a reliable means to determine compliance with hemodialysis.

Supply inventories: The use of materials required for home peritoneal dialysis during nursing home visits patients has been utilized at the University of Pittsburgh, USA, to compare compliant versus non-compliant patients. Forty-nine patients were investigated during home visits at three monthly intervals. Compliance was determined by percentages, and based upon the number of exchanges performed (based on inventory and deliveries), divided by the number of exchanges prescribed. The resultant percentage scored was considered in relationship to the following variables: staff evaluations, patient attitudes to compliance, demographics, hospitalizations, dialysis adequacy, 'Derogatis Affects Balance Sheet' (a validated tool of affects balance), and outcomes. Thirty Five percent of patients were found to be non-compliant with prescribed exchanges based upon the supply inventory. Age, race, gender, peritoneal dialysis time, and number of co-morbid conditions or incidence of diabetes could not differentiate Compliant and non-compliant patients. This method of evaluating compliance was found to be predictive of non-compliant behavior. Twenty-nine percent of non-compliant patients were changed to hemodialysis versus only 6 percent in case of compliant patients. The authors concluded that approximately one-third of the patients at their center did not comply with treatment, which in turn resulted in inadequate dialysis treatment and poor outcome (Bernardini & Piraino 1998).

Self-assessment: Self-assessment forms were used by researchers in Cleveland, USA, to determine patient's baseline functional health status in relationship to their clinical outcomes. The SF-36 score rating was used to assess baseline functional health status. The MOS SF-36 (Medical Outcome Study Short Form) is an adaptation of the full length MOS, a 36-question generic instrument without specific reference to chronic renal failure. The questions address the patient's ability to perform vigorous activity, daily activities and to participate in social, family and occupational activity. This scale is used to assess the patient's mood, current and past health and judges their energy and susceptibility to illness. The scales are scored on a 0 to 100 range; the higher number is a more favorable rating. The component summary scores combine the physical and mental of the eight scales into a physical and mental component summary score. One thousand patients were studied across three outpatient dialysis centers. The authors found that patients with physical component scores below the median were twice as likely to die and 1.5 times more likely to be hospitalized as patients with scores at or above the median score. In turn, patients who missed more than two treatments per month often had higher physical component score than patients who did not miss treatments (DeOreo 1997). In a recent study from Belgium, researchers tested a dialysis diet and fluid non-adherence questionnaire (DDFQ) in patients on hospital-based hemodialysis. Measuring weight gain, potassium and phosphate levels and serum albumin in patients who had non-compliant behaviors confirmed the validity of the questionnaire. They found that non-compliance with diet and fluid guidelines was very common, particularly in men and smokers. Younger age was also negatively correlated with non-adherence (Vlaminck et al. 2001).

Individual psychotherapeutic assessment: Psychologists at the University of Iowa, USA, hypothesized that there was a relationship between individual attentional style and compliance with medical regimen (Christensen et al. 1997). The authors focused on two attention styles in 51 patients with chronic renal disease in response to a 'health related threat'. Patients who were alert (high monitors) and those were ambivalent (low monitors) to harmful heath related factors. These researchers used the Miller Behavioral Styles Scale (MBSS) which assesses or 'monitors' individual attention styles in relationship to the patient's environment. Patients were asked to reconstruct in their mind four anxiety provoking scenarios, which was followed by questions as to how the patient would cope with such situations. In this study, patients considered to be high monitors were more likely to be active and alert to harmful health related factors versus patients considered to be low monitors.

SOCIO-DEMOGRAPHIC CHARACTERISTICS OF NON-COMPLIANT PATIENTS ON DIALYSIS

Socio-demographic characteristics such as race, age and length of time on hemodialysis of patients have been utilized in an attempt to predict compliance in hemodialysis patients (Leggat et al. 1998). In a study conducted in Ann Arbor, Michigan, USA, race, age, staff observations were used to predict non-compliance. They identified 6,251 patients who were on hemodialysis for more than one year. Non-compliance was defined in terms of missing one or more hemodialysis sessions in a month, shortening by ten or more minutes one or more sessions a month, an inter-dialytic dry weight gain of more than 5.7 percent, and serum phosphorus levels of greater than 7.5 mg/L. Overall 8.5 percent of patients missed hemodialysis sessions, 20 percent shortened their dialysis sessions (7 percent three or more times), 10 percent had more than 5.7 inter-dialytic dry weight gain, or serum phosphate of greater than 7.5 mg/L. Using the Cox proportional hazards models adjusted to incorporate the socio-demographic variables above, they found a significant correlation between non-compliance amongst blacks, patients between 20-39 years, and smokers. Amongst those who skipped one or more treatments a month, there was a 25 percent higher incidence of mortality; patients with greater than 5.7 percent inter-dialytic weight gain had a 35 percent higher incidence of mortality.

In a comparative study of male and female 'coping strategies' in two hemodialysis centers in the USA, 15 males and 15 females were surveyed retrospectively. The 'Jalowiec Coping Scale' was used to determine differences in coping strategies across the genders. This scale included 60 coping strategies and eight sub-scales and used a four point rating scale with zero indicating 'never used' and three indicating 'often used'. The eight coping styles in this scale are as follows: confrontative, evasive, optimistic, fatalistic, emotive, palliative, supportive and self-reliant. Findings suggested that both male and female patients tended to use emotionally focussed coping strategies (Blake 1996). The only significant variable to coping styles was determined by the number of years on hemodialysis, age, and degree of formal education. Patients on hemodialysis less than eight years, between the ages of 50-60 years, who had only undergone the mandatory formal education were more likely to use emotion-focused coping strategies.

In a later descriptive study from the United Kingdom, coping strategies of men receiving hemodialysis were once again examined. However, in this instance the authors attempted to conceptualize these strategies in relationship to a number of other social variables namely: their social networks, patient perceived social support, and conflict and reciprocity in their personal relationships. Thirty participants were studied using the 'Ways of Coping Questionnaire' and the 'Interpersonal Relationship Inventory'. The findings suggested that although both problem-focused and emotion-focused coping strategies were used, patients tended to use problem- focused coping, especially the seeking of social support. Overall, patients perceived high levels of social support and moderate to high levels of reciprocity with members of their social networks, and only moderate levels of conflict in their interpersonal relationships (Cormier-Daigle & Stewart 1997).

PSYCHOSOCIAL FACTORS INVOLVED IN NON-COMPLIANT PATIENTS ON DIALYSIS

Psychosocial factors have been considered in terms of non-compliant behavior and mortality in hemodialysis patients by a number of authors. In a prospective study at George Washington University Medical Center, USA, researchers attempted to determine the effects of psychosocial variables upon compliance with hemodialysis. Baseline or initial psychosocial variables of wellbeing in relationship to the effects of their illness and satisfaction with life were measured using the 'Beck Depression Inventory', serum albumin concentration, Kt/V and protein catabolic rate. Behavioral compliance was measured in terms of shortening of sessions and attendance. In addition, the type of hemodialyser was noted for each patient. Over a 26-month period it was found that lower levels of social support, decreased behavioral compliance with hemodialysis, and a negative perspective of the illness were associated with a significant increased risk of mortality (Sensky et al. 1996). This study served to emphasis the relationship between psychosocial wellbeing and compliance with hemodialysis. It emphasized the need for a positive perception of the illness and the need for social support in accepting the consequences of chronic illness.

Cognitive factors have also been combined with psychosocial variables to increase our understanding of compliance in patients receiving dialysis (Furr 1998). At the Charing Cross and Westminster Medical School, London, psychosocial and cognitive variables including gender, age, duration of time on hemodialysis, affective disturbance, past psychiatric history, health locus of control, social adjustments and social support of 45 patients in a single hemodialysis unit were measured using multiple regression analysis. Compliance was determined by adherence to diet (measured by pre-hemodialysis serum potassium), and to fluid restriction (inter-dialysis weight gain). The findings suggested that compliance was not significantly influenced by any one variable but by a complex interaction of all the above variables, thereby confirming the multi-factorial nature of non-compliance.

At the University of Iowa, USA, health beliefs and personality traits of individual hemodialysis patients were studied in relationship to compliance with the medical regime. The authors based their study on the hypothesis that the identification of pre-morbid conscious-type personality traits and beliefs would facilitate and ensure accurate prediction of patients' compliance with the medical regime. They used the 'Health Beliefs Model' and the 'Hierarchical Regression Analysis' to 70 patients on hemodialysis. They found that even those patients who were assessed to be conscientious and had appropriate health beliefs were found to be non-compliant with the hemodialysis regime. In this study, non-compliance was measured by inter-dialysis, weight gain, and serum phosphorous levels (Wiebe et al. 1997). These findings tend to suggest that the anxiety and stress of ongoing hemodialysis over rides pre-morbid conscientious-type traits, making the prediction of compliance unpredictable.

Fatigue is a common side effect found amongst hemodialysis patients and a recurring factor in those who do not comply adequately with treatment. In one study, 110 hemodialysis patients suffering from fatigue were studied to determine the relationship between fatigue, depressive mood, provision of social support, and biochemical data. Using a combination of fatigue scale, 'Beck Depression Inventory' and biochemical laboratory data, they found that although fatigue was relatively mild, there was a definitive correlation with depression (Chiang 1997).

NON-COMPLIANCE AMONGST RECIPIENTS OF KIDNEY TRANSPLANTS

The half-life of transplants has increased steadily, cadaver kidney transplants to 9-11 years and 15-17 years for living transplants. This has meant that each center is following larger numbers of transplants; in Glasgow we follow approximately 1700 recipients of adult kidney transplants. Current restrictions of health care financing does not allow each patient to be seen by a qualified therapist to address psychosocial concerns, some of these unresolved concerns may lead to non-compliance with medications. It is estimated that 25 percent of this cohort of patients may be non-compliance with medications; one-to-one therapy with a qualified therapist would be prohibitively expensive. In this scenario, we suggest that specific groups of patients be given special attention to increase the level of compliance such as younger, female, not married and non-Caucasians. Other specific patients groups who may require special attention are recipients of living transplants and were transplanted longer time ago with a history of previous transplant are also at risk of non-compliance. In addition, patients displaying emotional problems such as anxiety, hostility, depression, distress, lack of coping and avoidance behaviors may also be targeted for special attention by qualified therapists to increase medical compliance.

PRE-TRANSPLANT SCREENING

Pre-transplant screening should include psychosocial assessment using one or more of the standardized instruments to identify patients at risk of non-compliance after transplant. Although desirable, it is impossible to provide long-term counseling to all recipients of organ transplants. From this review, we conclude that patients who are at a higher risk of non-compliance after kidney transplants were younger, female, unmarried and non-Caucasians. Patients who were recipients of living transplants and were transplanted longer time ago with a history of previous transplant were also at risk of non-compliance. In general, all patients displaying emotional problems such as anxiety, hostility, depression, distress, lack of coping and avoidance behaviors were also at risk of non-compliance after kidney transplantation. A focused approach directed towards patients at high risk of non-compliance would be more cost effective. This strategy may decrease the number of kidney transplants lost due to non-compliance with resultant economic benefit to the society.

HOW DO WE MEASURE COMPLIANCE?

Kahan (2000) recently summarized the selection criteria for transplantation as follows: 'accepted notion of benefit' (medical need, life remaining and post-transplant quality of life); 'patient's rights' (based upon the right of every patient to transplantation is they so wish; 'cost effectiveness' (on the basis of best economic outcome); and 'scientific progress' (whether the patient's treatment will advance the medical science). These concepts are designed to assist the physician in allocating scarce resource of organs amongst an increasing number of patients. In general, psychosocial assessments have centered upon compliance, family support and the existence of any psychiatric disorders. Primary psychiatric contraindications generally include history of substance abuse, psychosis, suicide attempts, dementia and borderline personality. While 'soft' or as we feel should be more accurately quoted as subjective criteria, include obesity, mood disorder, legal history and family support. In the absence of a formalized assessment procedure, the transplant team is likely to rely upon the collective 'gut' instincts. 'Gut' instincts, however, are wholly inaccurate and unreliable as well as being unfair on both the patient and the staff. Such feelings can fluctuate from day to day with stress and personal circumstances and the society's prevailing norms which are likely to be biased against the minority and less educated members of the society.

The principal assessment tools include the Psychosocial Assessment of Candidates for Transplantation (PACT), the Psychosocial Levels System (PLS), and the Transplant Evaluating Rating Scale (TERS). The Beck Depression Inventory and Minnesota Multiphase Personality Inventory (MMPI) have also featured in a number of psychosocial studies amongst renal patients. PACT focuses upon psychological variables such as substance abuse, compliance, social support, psychopathology, lifestyle and knowledge of the transplant process. However, PACT does not predict transplant outcomes as such, rather it highlights the correlation between decisions to accept or exclude the view of different assessors between recipients.

The PLS evaluates the correlation of decisions to include or exclude patients, based upon past coping skills, psychiatric history, affect, mental health status, support and susceptibility to anxiety. Patients are subsequently classified into three levels of suitability for transplantation. Level One patients are characterized by not having any psychiatric history, appropriate social responses and good social support. Level Two patients are likely to have a history of depression, agitation or dysphoria and only satisfactory levels of social support at diagnosis. While those patients classified at Level three are liable to have a significant psychiatric history of substance abuse or major depression and/or suicidal ideation.

The TERS evaluates ten psychosocial aspects of a patients functioning and is an expansion of the PLS. In addition to the above-mentioned TERS, PLS level One candidates may display cluster C traits (avoidant, dependent or obsessive-compulsive personality disorders). Level Two patients may have cluster C traits or a combination of symptoms from clusters A (paranoid, schizoid, schizotypical personality disorders) and clusters B (anti social, borderline, histrionic, narcissistic personality disorder). Level Three candidates have cluster A and B diagnosis. The use of the above mentioned assessments have been aimed at the development a single or multiple measure of psychosocial suitability for transplantation, the underlining criteria being whether or not the patient would be likely or capable of complying with the post-transplant regime. However, despite the use of rating tools, there is little consensus about the most effective method of predicting outcome. While other disparities center around the emphasis placed on any number of psychosocial factors and the validity of predicting post-transplant behavior based on past performance. Despite studies which have suggested that it is becoming increasingly difficult to predict patient outcome there remains a dogged reliance upon such scales and assessments, which utilize psychiatric classifications. Therefore, one might argue that the ability to predict compliance behavior is only as good as the initial diagnosis. Therefore, in our view we feel that they tend not to offer any further insight into patient's psychosocial or transpersonal worlds and patients are typified or classified at the time of assessment, not allowing for any future shift in position.

We are particularly concerned that chronic illness might exaggerate or underplay particular traits (consistent behavior) or states (two or more traits) and the subsequent psychological profile (two or more states). This would make an accurate assessment difficult and may obscure how a person might behave if relatively well (after a transplant) as opposed to relative unwell (before a transplant) near impossible. It may well determine how a patient is functioning on the day of the test, but not over time leading to an inaccurate test result. Upon reflection, such assessments are incongruent with contemporary psychotherapeutic input, which considers patient experience in terms of a dynamic and interactive 'process' of change and personal development. Any assessment should take into account the effect upon the individual-self, defined in terms of autonomy, identity, individuality, liberty, choice and fulfillment of ongoing chronic illness. There is also the authenticity of the patient's presentation to consider, while interacting with a staff member they may feel hesitant and nervous. Therefore, they might present with the best case scenario usually accompanied by a tendency towards politeness and reservation than they ordinarily would present. Therefore, a 'one off' scale might not have the accuracy and insight of a psychotherapeutic profile which, is built up over a number of sessions when patients might be more at ease with themselves.

Generally speaking, patients receiving dialysis or kidney transplants often present in our clinic as in the form of a 'challenged' self, whereby their fundamental guiding emotional resources and identity which have served them pre-morbidly, have shifted in keeping with the course of their illness. Transplant patients are at a disadvantage when being assessed by the instruments, which have as their baseline a sense of individual equilibrium or normality. Everyday normality or reality for renal patients is different to that of non-renal patients. Renal patients live in a world which is unpredictable, uncertain and where daily living is geared towards their survival' or a dynamic, responsive process as opposed to the static existence depicted in assessment tools. We consider the former to be much more apt in a psychosocial research environment where increasingly, human development is compared to a human cell, with surrounding membrane to determine the 'edge' where the individual ends and the external environment begins, commonly referred to as emotional boundaries.

We often find themselves in the role of witness and ally (as patients relive their experiences), in whose presence they can speak the unspeakable and think the unthinkable. This work is not for the faint hearted, as he/she will need to utilize any flair for the 'transliterate prose' referred to in the previous chapter as a means to build bridges between the patients and staff. In the face of barely veiled antagonism from other members of the transplant team, it will be the therapist's confidence and clinical judgment that will sustain them through treatment sessions. In the name of good practice, and to ensure that others understand our work, we have developed a systematic model of psychotherapeutic profiling in place of standardized instruments in a move towards inclusion, as opposed to exclusion from the transplant process. This ensures that a holistic picture of the patient is presented at various points in their lives and allows staff to better understand their presentation and enables us to intervene in times of crisis in a more informed manner.

When administering scales and assessments with a view to screening patients for suitability for transplantation, mental health professionals need to convey to the patient the nature of their primary role. This is particularly important not only for the patient but the mental health professional as there is potential for abuse of our professional expertise. Mental health professionals might want to consider whether they want to be perceived by patients as assessing their emotional wellbeing with a view to supporting and working towards the resolution of their problems or as a means to gain information for the purpose of excluding them from the transplant process. If mental health professionals do not declare their empathy, then they might be considered by patients as underhand and as a profession to be feared and engaged with in a cautious manner. We have often come across this attitude amongst patients when we have approached them to make them aware of the psychotherapy service after they have received their yearly medical assessment for the purpose of staying on the transplant list while on dialysis. Consequently, it is often difficult to determine the severity of the emotional suffering amongst these patients and any potential for support and intervention.

Given the traditional role of mental health professionals (especially psychiatrists and psychologists in particular), it is hardly surprising that patient skepticism is one of the major obstacles to treatment. One can hardly expect a patient to share his/her intimate thoughts and concerns with us if they are uncertain as to how we might utilize this information. It is our belief that mental health professionals working with transplant patients or any other field of chronic illness should not be regarded merely as gatekeepers, but rather as a part of a team.

PSYCHOTHERAPEUTIC PERSPECTIVE OF NON-COMPLIANCE

As the reader would have deduced from the chapter so far, studies of compliance behavior have been founded upon demographic and psychological variables aimed at predicting compliance or to include, exclude or 'select' patients from the transplant list. However, such psychological and demographic variables are not only conflicting, but serve to maneuver groups of patients into homogenous, high risk or 'vulnerable' classifications without consideration of their individual social, emotional or environmental circumstances. Further, if implemented rigidly in assessment clinics, whole sections of the community are likely to be excluded from transplant programs. For example, patients who unwittingly fall into a high-risk categorization (e.g. black females from low socio-economic groups) are at best likely to be viewed with some skepticism. Therefore, it is probably fair to conclude that such research is of little clinical relevance to the practicing physician in the transplant clinic.

Latterly, there has been an increasing trend amongst studies towards the contemplation of non-compliance as a less tangible, conscious phenomenon (Cramer 1995 & 1999, Baines & Jindal 2001). Most notably, non-compliance manifests as missed clinic appointments and drug 'holidays'. We have interpreted these actions as a more independent behavioral pattern as they move away from the perception of themselves as ill. When contemplating such non-compliance retrospectively (after graft loss), patients often view such manifestations in terms of personal development or progression (away from their perception of themselves as being ill) as opposed to regression or being non-compliant with the post-transplant regime. In contrast, the conscious acknowledgement of the ongoing need for compliance with immunosuppressive medication is synonymous with the realization that all patients retain the potential for relapse, despite having received a successful transplant. Traditionally, the patient's perspective of non-compliance has been considered in terms of the extent of the 'denial' of their illness and failure to adjust to the stringency of the medical regime, alone with the 'intrinsic strength' and their ability to 'cope'. Also, they are often penalized for being unemployed despite research which has showed that patients on dialysis have difficulty in maintaining paid work, due to feelings of lethargy, prejudice of employers and the impingement of dialysis in their work place.

PSYCHOTHERAPEUTIC PROFILING OF NON-COMPLIANT PATIENTS

The above mentioned scales and instruments are often known in the business as *psychological* profiling, a collection of data pertaining to an individual or group from a formal test. This data is then utilized as means to predict behavior and/or typify an individual's personality. Mental health professionals have utilized this to classify patients into traits. Employers and investigative agencies use this data to predict how she or he may behave or perform in particular situations. However, patients presenting for transplantation are for the most part not career mental health patients, potential employees or dangerous criminals; they are human beings who have to confront with their own existential reality or mortality somewhat prematurely. Rather than considering patients in terms of traits, we prefer to consider them in terms of multi-faceted personas that may or may not respond to experiences and situations in a predictable manner. While transplantation is not the panacea for all their health problems and in itself carries medical risk, it is for these patients, their only chance. Renal patients have a different 'ontic' and 'ontological' reality to non-dialysis/transplant patients; their baseline of normality and reality is different to their contemporaries. Therefore, we have set about giving our patients the best chance of inclusion through personal development and ongoing support.

Psychotherapeutic profiling as defined by us is collected over a period of time (up to twelve sessions) and resists classifying patients into traits or typifying personality types. Rather, we prefer to consider them from a more plural perspective or series of sub personalities that in different circumstances and presented with different dilemmas will interact with each other to produce a different self. Furthermore, psychotherapeutic profiling is not considered purely the domain of the therapist but is formed in collaboration with the patient. The ensuing insight will enable the patient to better understand his/her behavior and change it; the therapist will be best placed to assist the patient to implement change. Our work is based upon the belief that non-compliant patients have the potential to produce a shift in their behavior if they have more insight into it and feel supported and understood. Also unlike psychological profiling, psychotherapeutic profiling in this context is not a static intrusive and conclusive tool, but a dynamic collaborative means with potential for intervention. In addition, it can be used insightfully to plan other supportive services and medical treatment regimes so that they best serve the needs of the patients.

Developing psychotherapeutic profiling: The protocol for psychotherapeutic profiling was initially formulated, refined and developed upon our work with 25 post-transplant patients (11 women, 14 men) who were non-compliant with dialysis who subsequently received a kidney transplant. These patients went on to comply with the post-transplant regime. Subsequently, these principles and pattern of intervention have been applied to all such patients that have come through our program. The first 25 patients were referred to psychotherapy within three months of receiving a kidney transplant. While each individual experience was different; common presenting symptoms were feelings of guilt after receiving a kidney from a cadaver source, fear and confusion about their own potential for non-compliance, low mood, anxiety and hesitancy regarding the future. All 25 patients underwent a 12-week course of time-sensitive individual Systemic Integrative Psychotherapy (Baines & Jindal 2000).

Patients in this study complied (measured in terms of keeping clinic appointments, attendance at psychotherapy sessions and medications) with the post-transplant regime, despite being non-compliant with hemodialysis. This cohort of patients was characterized by unremarkable psychological histories prior to hemodialysis and had maintained some social contact with friends or family throughout dialysis.

Dialysis was found to trigger a mood state of negative feelings, defensive and motivational behavior that could be directly traced through therapy to an 'internalization' of a pre-morbid relationship, most notably, the loss of a parent during childhood or a childhood experience of being different, that became 'externalized' in the present. Therefore, dialysis became the object of transference that was subsequently 'internalized' along with the self. Non-compliance was seen as a means to differentiate oneself from the earlier pre-morbid state. The role of the therapist was to identify the pre-morbid mood and contextualize it in the present, as a means to facilitate patient insight into their non-compliant behavior. Patient insight regarding their earlier non-compliant behavior was accompanied by a reduction in fear as to their future potential towards non-compliance with the post-transplant regime. All patients reported a decrease in low mood, guilt, anxiety and insomnia after completion of the full course of therapy. However, long- term follow up will be necessary to see if these patients maintain their emotional wellbeing and medical compliance.

STRATEGIES TO INCREASE COMPLIANCE

Patient empowerment: There is an increasing trend to involve patients directly in treatment planning which in turn may lead to increased compliance with dialysis. A number of surveys have indicated that patients would like more control over the non-technical aspects of dialysis (Montemuro et al. 1994). There is clearly a need to increase patient participation in all aspects of their disease process. However, there has been little legislative support for this position (in the United Kingdom, patients do not have a right to choose their physician or hospital of treatment) and little detail as to how staff coax patients towards the communicative and behavioral competence necessary for meaningful empowerment. Empowerment does not come about by some miraculous process of osmosis but through the acquisition of communicative and behavioral competence on the part of both the staff and the patient. Skills, which may well, be lacking amongst patients from lower socio-economic groups who might be easily overwhelmed by the professional classes and/or whose confidence and self-esteem have been eroded by chronic illness. These patients will need to be presented with empowerment as a multi-component educational package that may utilize modeling, coaching, feedback and homework assignments, all conducted within a supportive and developmental framework.

To date, empowerment studies have been predominantly concerned with the more compliant and/or independent patient. However, within the supportive and educational framework the more non-compliant patient might also be considered. Many of the non-compliant or emotionally traumatized patients featured in this book have developed such a presentation in part, because their personalities are such that they do not perform well within a rigid structured hospital environment. Therefore, they may respond better within the semi-structured framework of a patient empowerment program. In contrast, previously compliant patients who might appear to be seemingly obvious candidates for such a program might not do so well in the semi-structured, self-initiating, empowered environment. In short, empowerment programs should be viewed as an ongoing system of personal development, education and support, with patient being selected on a case-by-case basis.

In a recent study aimed at the retrospective determination of compliance with medications amongst patients who had experienced late acute rejection, we requested that they complete a modified version of the Long-term Medication Behavior Self-efficacy Scale (LTMBS-scale) a self-report questionnaire (Baines et al. 2002). The questionnaire, which they were able to complete in their own time, was aimed at determining patient's levels of confidence in taking their medications in a variety of environmental and situational contexts and with a view to offering supportive psychotherapeutic intervention. In the spirit of self-empowerment, the questionnaire was not 'administered' by the physician; rather the statements were aimed to prompt introspection and contemplation of individual patient circumstances and experiences thought to be vital in determining compliance behavior.

We retrospectively analyzed the case records of patients who had their first cadaver renal transplantation at our center during a six-year period from January 1991 to December 1996. We identified 26 patients who had late acute rejection. All patients received similar anti-rejection therapy. The Long-term Medication Behavior self-efficacy Scale is a 27-item instrument depicting a variety of situations in which the patient might be required to take their medication. The self-efficacy score was calculated by summing the scores of all items divided by 27. Thus the self-efficacy scores range between 1 and 3; higher score indicates greater self-efficacy. We modified the original scale to a 3-point questionnaire as our pilot study showed that patients found it difficult to discriminate between 5 options. Over a six-year period, we identified 26 patients with late acute rejection, two had subsequently died. The questionnaire was mailed to the remaining 24 patients (14 women and 10 men), with an explanatory letter; patients were requested to complete the questionnaire anonymously. After two weeks, we called each patient to inquire if they had completed the questionnaire. If the response was negative, we encouraged patients to complete and return the questionnaire. Confidence of each patient was computed by summing up all the responses and dividing by 27. The values range from 1 (least confident) to 3 (most confident). When a comparison of clinical data was needed, t-test was used. Statistical significance was assumed at a p value of 0.05. The mean values are expressed as mean +/- standard deviation. For statistical analysis and construction of the graph, a software package (SPSS 9, SPSS inc. Chicago) was used.

Our overall results showed a definitive correlation between late acute rejection, and individual patient's perceived low rate of self-efficacy across a variety of contextual or environmental situations. It was seen that patients were only reasonably confident (mean score 2.17) in taking their medication in the above-mentioned contexts. All patients demonstrated significantly lower self-efficacy in relationship to items 14, 20 and 21 (mean score 1.0), the items relating to physical and psychological symptoms (brittle bones and generally feeling 'very ill') and psychological symptoms (feeling 'sad') that affected their wellbeing. These symptoms were considered to be side effects of either the medications or a response to the experience of chronic illness.

The majority of patients (10 women, 5 men) returned their completed questionnaires before the two-week telephone reminder. However, the seven questionnaires (4 women, 3 men) that were returned after the telephone reminder demonstrated an even lower self-efficacy score (mean score 1.2). The second group of patients demonstrated the same trends in relationship to items 14, 20 and 21 as with the first group of patient (who returned their questionnaire without prompting), self-efficacy scores were significantly reduced for these items as well (mean score 0.5).

The overall results of the study suggested that patients were not confident that they would take their medication if they were liable to experience physical (brittle bones, generally feeling ill) and psychological (feelings of sadness) side effects of medication. These negative physical and psychological states were related to low self-efficacy with the taking of immunosuppressive medications and subsequent non-compliance. In addition, the ongoing nature of the symptoms served to maintain their perspective of themselves as 'ill' and therefore different from non-transplant patients or their peers, family and the general population. Of the patients who received supportive psychotherapy before receiving a second transplant, the aims of treatment were constructed around a shift in patient's ability to tolerate their individual difference (the need to take medications for their lifetime), in relationship to the majority of the population. This was achieved through the utilization of empowerment techniques such as modeling, systematic desensitization (gradual exposure) and homework assignments.

Items used in the questionnaire to study correlation between non-compliance and late acute rejection

1. At home
2. Pills are large and difficult to swallow
3. If medicine is expensive
4. If medication aids arc absent
5. Nobody helps to get ready
6. While at work
7. In a weekend
8. If medicine can make one impotent (male) or decrease interest in sex (female)
9. If the medicine can cause spots on face and excessive hair growth
10. Feeling healthy
11. Alternate day medications
12. The time for taking medicines do not coincide with meals
13. Doing a project at home
14. If medicines give brittle bones
15. If no one reminds of the time to take the medicine
16. When there are visitors at home
17. If angry at a friend
18. If in pain
19. While watching an exciting program in TV
20. Feeling ill
21. If feeling sad
22. When unknown people are watching (like in a restaurant)
23. If sick in stomach
24. If had an argument with the partner
25. At a party
26. While taking a long walk
27. In a bar

Formal Counseling: Dialysis results in inevitable changes in life-style and it is not uncommon for patients to become depressed in response to the loss of their pre-morbid lifestyle and anxious about their present and future well-being. This more so if they have a pre-morbid history of mental illness (Craven & Farrow 1993, Katayama & Kodama 1994, Drummond-Young et al. 1996, Abbey & Farrow, 1998). A common means to address depression and anxiety in this group of patients is to implement counseling and psychotherapy programs. The renal and transplant center at the University of Toronto, Canada, has successfully implemented a comprehensive counseling and psychotherapy program aimed at facilitating the adjustment of organ (liver, kidney, heart and lung) transplant patients, while supporting them through psychosocial and psychiatric support. To support, patients on dialysis and awaiting kidney transplants the 'While you are waiting' psycho-educational group was formed which comprised of a support and educational program. Group discussions involved living with a life threatening illness, preparing to live versus preparing to die, and preparing for transplantation (Abbey & Farrow 1998). However, while beneficial to relatively emotionally stabile patients, in keeping with position in the previous chapter, it should be remembered that the 'group' work of Abbey & Farrow (1998) placed emphasis upon education and support. They did not describe a group psychotherapeutic process or alliance and therefore should not be considered or directly compared with the findings from psychotherapy group studies, which are aimed at more emotionally volatile patients and which described a psychotherapeutic alliance and process.

At the University of North Carolina, USA, cognitive behavioral counseling was combined with stress inoculation education in an attempt to reduce anxiety, depression, adjustment to illness, stress and increase compliance to dialysis (Courts 1991). Psychosocial reactions and adherence to the medical regime, interpersonal support, and control, were identified as the intervening variables. The variables were founded on the pre-determined belief that while the physiological aspects of hemodialysis were well documented the psychosocial reaction to them would be 'unique'. Psychosocial change was measured using an assortment or though not necessarily compatible set of scales including: Clinical Anxiety Scale, Generalized Contentment Scale, Psychosocial Adjustment to Illness Scale Self-Report, and the

Hemodialysis Adjustment to Illness Scale. The findings suggested that a significant number of patients benefited from both cognitive behavioral counseling and the stress inoculation counseling; all patients demonstrated a lower post-test anxiety scores. More specifically, four patients had significantly reduced their pre-test depression scores and three had lower perceptions of dialysis stresses. Overall, four out of six patients had a higher post-test adjustment to illness score.

Multi-Disciplinary Approach: Adhering to an appropriate and adequate diet while on dialysis has been emphasized in a number of studies, as these patients are at a particular risk of malnutrition (DeOreo 1997). At the University Dialysis Center, Syracuse, USA, dieticians and physical therapists combined physical exercise and dietary recommendations to assess nutritional intake in relationship to patient participation in an intra-dialytic exercise program (DeOreo 1997). Performance testing and nutrition assessments were administered to 16 patients who participated in a self-paced intra-dialytic exercise program, which included cycling before or during dialysis. Baseline data was collected pre-dialysis, and at 3, 6, and 12 month intervals. After 12 months, patients demonstrated significant improvements in physical and nutritional wellbeing, which in turn was directly related to compliance with dialysis. The role of the social worker amongst dialysis patients has not received much attention. However, one study gave particular emphasis to psychosocial problems as obstacles to compliance with dialysis. Compliance was discussed with reference to the life cycle stage of the patient; elderly and younger patients more likely to be non-compliant. This study emphasized the impact of psychosocial environment of the patient as a critical determinant in ensuring compliance (Furr 1998).

Complementary Medicine: This form of therapy does not readily lend itself to traditional research methodology, and therefore, it has been suggested that its effectiveness has not been clearly demonstrated. Despite some misgivings, complementary therapy has been incorporated into traditional medical treatment in a wide range of specialties including midwifery (Botting 1998), oncology (Howells & Maher1998), and coronary care patients (Ai et al. 1997). In a study amongst coronary artery bypass patients at the University of Michigan, USA, complementary therapies have been used to promote psychological recovery, post-surgical anxiety and depression (Ai et al.

1997). Complementary therapies were used successfully to alleviate pain, promote relaxation, and facilitate adjustment to lifestyle changes and as a means to allowing patients some participatory control over their illness and recovery. The parallels between coronary care bypass patients and our patients, such as the ongoing lethargy in response to a disease process, vulnerability to depression and anxiety, and the need for a change in lifestyle, suggest that these forms of therapy may well be beneficial.

Conclusion

Non-compliance with dialysis is not necessarily an accurate predictor of post-transplant compliance and should not always be used to exclude patients from the transplant program. However, patients with a history of non-compliance with dialysis are liable to feelings of fear of a recurrence of non-compliance behavior which might jeopardize their kidney transplant, but over which they feel they have no control. They may have symptoms of anxiety, insomnia, guilt at having received a kidney from a cadaver source, hesitancy regarding the future and low mood. These mood states can be effectively treated using short-term psychotherapy aimed at increased understanding of past non-compliant behavior. In turn, such insight creates a more stable and productive mood state and facilitates actualization of a better quality of life in the future.

The treatment of non-compliance has been fragmented and lacks uniformity with regards to the identification and prediction of treatment policy. Ultimately, the transplant community needs an inclusive model of compliance capable of detecting and treating non-compliance before it proves fatal. It is hoped that our work will encourage others towards a multi-faceted approach using psychotherapeutic principles as a means to detect, understand and treat this condition in patients on dialysis and in recipients of kidney transplants.

Chapter 10:

Anxiety and Depression in Patients Receiving Dialysis and Kidney Transplantation

RE: Munesh
From: Anita Cumbermack
Sent: Fri 9/05/08 5:21 PM
To: rahul jindal
Cc: Kamela Bemaul; Ryhan Singh

Hello,

I spoke with Munesh and mom today - they deny any depressed feelings. Mom has indicated family problems (differences).

Latest labs:
Creat = 2.6
Na = 144.7
K = 3.48
Cl = 111.5
Ca = 7.2
Phos = 5.2
FBS = 84 mg/dl
Urine proteins – trace
Pus = 2 in 12HPF
Bacteria +/HPF

Will repeat his labs on Sunday.

Anita Florendo-Cumbermack, MD
Medical Officer, Department of Medicine, GPHC,
Georgetown, Guyana

RE: munesh
From: Anita Cumbermack
Sent: Mon 9/08/08 7:59 PM
To: rahul jindal; Ravi, Asha Purohit
Cc: Kamela Bemaul; Ryhan Singh

BUN = 2.3
Creat = 38
Ca = 6.8
Phos = 5.3
Hb = 8.1
WBC = 6,300
P = 81
L = 17
E = 2
Plt = 392,000
Retic = 1.5

There seems to be an issue with his mother—She kept calling me and telling me she's getting pain and when I arrange for her to be seen she either doesn't show up or becomes abusive with staff. I will try to arrange a meeting with her and some counseling.

Also wanted to let you know that I will be handing over the duty of correspondence and patient interaction to Drs. Ryhan Singh and Kamela Bemaul. I will however e-mail the patient information to you before I leave. We also spoke with Mr. Khan who will organize the renal angiograms.

Unable to get CMV testing done, working on urine creatinines.

Anita Florendo-Cumbermack
Medical Officer, Department of Medicine, GPHC,
Georgetown, Guyana

Anxiety in patients receiving dialysis and kidney transplants is much more complex and multifaceted than originally thought. There is a notable absence of prospective long-term or longitudinal studies looking at the specific clinical manifestation of anxiety (post-traumatic stress disorder, obsessive-compulsive disorder and phobias) and depression in patients receiving dialysis and kidney transplantation. Psychological intervention to address these disorders in dialysis or transplant patients has been intermittent. However, those that have monitored intervention, suggest that patients need timely and precise psychological attention both before and after transplant. Furthermore, this intervention needs to be sensitive to numerous issues, such as relationship conflict, hope, uncertainty, fear, spirituality and guilt all of which correlate to depression and anxiety.

Anxiety and depression in patients receiving dialysis and kidney transplants is increasingly being recognized as an important problem. The incidence of anxiety, depression and other psychiatric disorders in hospitalized patients with end-stage renal disease was analyzed in a cohort study of Medicare dialysis patients (Kimmel 1998). The results suggested that 9 percent of all hospitalized end-stage renal disease patients in the study were admitted with a diagnosis of depression, anxiety, alcohol and drug abuse. Further, men, African-Americans, and younger patients were significantly more likely to be hospitalized. Given that depression and anxiety is not uncommon amongst dialysis patients there has been concern to determine whether rate of hospitalizations and mortality can be predicted by physicians of the basis of depressive symptoms and patient self-report instruments. Data from the Dialysis Outcomes and Practice Patterns Study (DOPPS), which randomly analyzed 2855 hemodialysis (HD) patients across 142 facilities in the United States and 2401 patients from 101 facilities from Europe, identified all patients with a documented diagnosis of depression in their medical records (Lopes 2002). In addition, patients were asked to complete two self-report questions pertaining to their mood in the four weeks leading up to the project as follows; *'so down in the dumps that nothing could cheer you up'* and secondly *'downhearted and blue.'* The results indicated that overall there was a 20 percent prevalence of depression. The self-report questionnaire showed an increased risk of mortality and hospitalization amongst HD patients.

While anxiety has been shown repeatedly to be one of a cluster of symptoms amongst dialysis patients (Yeh 2004), anxiety has also been shown to rise within two months of transplantation by as much as 25 percent (Watnick 2003), an increase attributed to the anxiety and stress of undergoing transplantation. In a cross sectional study of twenty male and twenty female transplant patients were assessed using BDI, Hospital Anxiety Depression Scales (HADS), Speilberger Trait Anxiety Inventory (STAI-I) and Beck Hopeless Scale (BHS) (Watnick 2003). Major depressive episodes were observed in 25 percent of patients, with individual patient variables such as age, gender, education, marital status, income, type of transplant, did not vary significantly between patients with or without depression. In a group of fifty patients with End Stage Renal Failure (ESRD), investigators used Beck's Depression Inventory (BDI), Illness Effects Questionnaire, Multi-dimensional Scales of Social Support and Satisfaction with Life Scale Results. They found that depression was significant (Power 2002). Further, when compared to ESRD patients who had just started HD, the level of perceived social support was significantly less. The overall conclusions suggested that greater the negative perception of illness, the patient is to more likely to be depressed and have lower Quality of Life (QOL). It also seems that there is a need for greater social support amongst patients with ESRD.

However, there have been suggestions that over the longer term, anxiety is less evident in transplant patients than their dialysis counterparts (Procci 1980). In a comparative study of thirty-two males, sixteen undergoing maintenance HD and sixteen who had received a cadaver kidney transplant, social disability, including depression and sexual dysfunction, was measured using the Ruesch Social Disability Rating Scale. Both groups experienced similar levels of social disability and interference with their pre-morbid lifestyle. Indeed, social disability was more likely to be determined by socio-economic variables such as whether or not the patient was employed, financial stability and degree of depression and sexual functioning.

Depression amongst HD patients has also been linked to withdrawal from dialysis and death (McDade-Montez 2006). Two hundred and forty HD patients participated in a longtitudinal study over a period of four years after having been diagnosed with depression. Of these, 18 percent withdrew from dialysis treatment with symptoms of depression, being determined by multivariate survival analysis, seen as a significant risk factor.

Anxiety in Relationship to Quality of Life

Depression, anxiety and adjustment to illness have been contemplated in terms of QOL, with QOL thought to be higher amongst Peritoneal Dialysis (PD) compared to HD patients (Diaz-Buxo 2000), but overall much higher amongst transplant patients, despite them still being liable to anxiety and depression (Overbeck 2005). In a comparative study, SF-36 was used to evaluate the QOL of 16,755 HD and 1260 PD patients. Patients on PD tended to be younger, white, with lesser incidence of diabetes, lower albumin concentrations, and higher creatinine, hemoglobin and white blood cell counts (Diaz-Buxo 2000). The findings suggested that while the two groups of patients had similar levels of physical functioning, patients on PD scored better in terms of emotional well-being and had adjusted better to their illness in terms of been less disruption to their daily lives.

In a cross-sectional study, QOL was compared in 76 renal transplant patients and patients with ESRD and who were awaiting a transplant (Overbeck 2005). Both groups were asked to assess their quality of life using the BDI, the State-Trait Anxiety Inventory (STAI) and the Psychological Adjustment to Illness Scale (PAIS). The results suggested that the socio-demographic and general health perception were similar between both groups, physical functioning amongst the transplant patients was significantly higher both groups. However, unemployment remains high amongst both groups. The ongoing negative, disabling effects that ongoing chronic illness can have upon HRQL and mood have also been considered in terms of compliance behavior using BDI and Beck Anxiety Inventory (BAI), the SF-36 and The Kidney Transplant Questionnaire (Covic 2004).

Anxiety and Depression in Relationship to Non-Adherence

In a systematic review of the literature on medical non-adherence after kidney transplantation in the cyclosporine era, common variables that may help the clinician in early intervention were identified (Jindal 2003). Common variables rendering patients a higher risk to non-compliance were younger, female, unmarried and non-Caucasians. The authors also found that patients experiencing emotional problems such as anxiety and depression were equated with poor coping and avoidant type behaviors. Indeed, non-adherent patients showed greater emotional distress, higher transplant-related stress, lack of control over their treatment process in terms of medications, as well as, little perceived control over transplant outcome and higher situational-operational knowledge.

Negative correlations between physical functioning and mental status have been reported and considered further in terms of adherence with immunosuppressant medication (Goetzmann 2006). In a multi-organ study that included ninety-eight heart, lung, liver and kidney transplant recipients, subjective and cognitive experiences of taking immunosuppressants was measured, before and at twelve months follow up. Patients were assessed using multiple scales, including Sense of Coherence (SOC), Hospital Anxiety and Depression Scale (HADS-D), SF-36, Satisfaction with Life, Medication Experience Scale for Immunosuppressants and Social Support. The treating physicians also assessed adherence with medications. Twelve months post-transplant there were significant negative correlations between physical functioning, mental health status, satisfaction with life and social support. However, there were also significant negative correlations between pre- and post-transplant adherence behavior. In addition, the authors suggested that the MESI emerged as an effective screening instrument for recording the cognitive and subjective attitudes of patients towards their immunosuppressant medication.

Discussion

Depression and anxiety appear to manifest during HD and persists, albeit to a lesser extent, after organ transplant (Sensky 1989; Haq 1991). Out of fifty-one patients on HD who were subjected to a standardized psychiatric interview, 33 percent were found to have classifiable anxiety and depression issues. Patients with a pre-morbid psychiatric history were more likely to experience psychological problems and require a psychiatric follow during follow up. The incidence of psychiatric disorders dropped to 17 percent following transplant. In a further study, an equal number of dialysis and transplant patients were subjected to a Socio-Psychiatric-Profile. Analysis of the profiles using the Bender Gestalt Scale suggested that dialysis patients were more likely to be diagnosed with anxiety and depression than their transplanted counterparts; normal status amongst transplant patients was significantly higher for depression and anxiety.

Specific psychosocial variables, including race, lower rate of patient perceived QOL and not having any previous acquaintances amongst dialysis patients, tend to render some patients more liable to depression than others, particularly during the first few months of dialysis. In a multicenter prospective cohort study, 123 patients were interviewed within ten days of starting their dialysis regime. The Beck Depression Inventory was used to assess depressive symptoms and found that 44 percent of the patients were classifiable as suffering from a major depressive episode and a further 21 percent were found to have lesser or mild symptoms of depression. Patients that were Caucasian, had a lower self-rated QOL, and no previous acquaintances receiving dialysis, were more likely to be depressed. Further, only 16 percent of patients classified as suffering from a major depressive episode and 13 percent of those with mild depressive symptoms were found to be receiving psychological intervention.

Comparative studies of HD and PD patients have considered anxiety and adjustment to illness using the Short Form 36 (SF 36) [Diaz-Buxo 2000]. Generalized anxiety disorder was analyzed in relationship to adjustment to illness in a group of 102 dialysis patients, fifty-eight kidney transplant patients and forty-two general anxiety patients. While patients with generalized anxiety disorder were found to have the highest number of depressive and anxiety symptoms, patients on dialysis had a high rate of psychiatric morbidity and a low rate of psychological intervention. Using the BDI, 47 percent of the sixty dialysis patients sampled were found to be depressed and exhibited suicidal intentions suggesting that regular psychological screening of these patients was necessary and that timely intervention could improve patient outcomes.

1. Causes of Anxiety and Depression in Patients Receiving Dialysis and Kidney Transplantation

Anxiety and depression in dialysis and renal transplant patients has been attributed to a number of factors including the negative side effects of immunosuppressant medication, adjustment to illness, non-adherence, dysfunctional body image and uncertainty. However, a successful transplant and subsequent potential for improved mental status, enhanced QOL, the re-establishment of some normality has been considered a motivating factor in patients who elect for organ transplant. However, post-transplant, stress and anxiety associated with the negative side-effects of immunosuppressant medications which include pain, weakness, fatigue, weight gain, facial changes and their negative impact upon patient's mental status has been a concern for some time (Perez-San-Gregoria 2005; Rosenberger 2005).

High personal control over the dialysis process has been associated with less psychiatric morbidity. The negative impact of illness upon patient's personal life has also been demonstrated to be considerably less. Eighty-two patients on HD completed the SF-36 and the Revised Illness Perception Questionnaire. The results suggest that there is a relationship between low QOL, perception of control and evidence of anxiety and depression. Personal higher control over their illness was associated with a lower emotional response (Cvengros 2004).

The psychological impact of the intrusiveness of ongoing dialysis and organ transplant is thought to contribute to anxiety and depression. Thirty-five HD, ten PD and twenty-five post-transplant patients participated in a standardized, self-report measure of negative and positive mood including, life happiness, self esteem, depression, anxiety and somatic symptoms of distress. The results were further correlated in terms of age, general health and their levels of defensiveness. The findings supported previous findings that negative mood and low perceptions of control over their illness were equated with high levels of psychological distress, poor adjustment to illness and repeated hospital admissions.

The relationship between adjustment to illness and Generalized Anxiety Disorder (GAD) in terms of dialysis and kidney transplant patients has gained increased attention over the last few years. This has been generated as a result of studies that have suggested that there is a link between GAD and ongoing unemployment or occupational disability, a significant problem amongst post-transplant patients.

The psychological status of the patient runs parallel with the course of the illness, with psychological intervention beginning at the pre-operative stage. Other investigators have preferred to profile patients, a process which runs parallel to the course of the illness and provides a basis for intervention. Such studies need to be coupled with intervention as these patients do respond. Early living donor studies have equated anxiety with donors, and more recently with recipients. Recipients are no longer being portrayed as willing to take an organ from a relative irrespective of the psychological status of the relationship. Indeed, recipients are able to discriminate between suitable and unsuitable donors.

Anxiety provoking thoughts regarding body image have also been reported amongst patients who received successful transplants from unknown donors.

2. Psychological Intervention

Psychologists working with renal patients have formulated a step-by-step intervention program for patients presenting with a heightened sense or fear of rejection after transplantation. The framework is focused upon identify points of certainty within the patient's life, starting with the treatment environment. It has been suggested that the concept of certainty has been considered from a psychosocial perspective. The authors use step-by-step interventions to create certainty within the patient's life and more importantly security within the psychotherapeutic alliance. The introduction of certainty and security may also give way to an element of control over the disease process on the part of the patient.

Other psychologists working amongst dialysis patients have observed anorexia nervosa in both males and females which correlated to anxiety, centered around fluid intake in relationship to the body's changing shape as opposed to weight. This phenomenon was seen by the patients as an opportunity to impose control over the disease process at the expense of adherence to fluid intake. The authors also urged psychologists to consider treating eating disorders in renal patients existentially as opposed to the treatment of choice, CBT, which, they argue parallels dialysis in that it is a rigid and uncompromising regime, and may cause the patient to become more entrenched in their non-adherent, controlled position.

Consultation liaison psychiatrists involved in pre-transplant consultation suggest that the psychiatric presentation of dialysis patients differ from regular liaison consults. While dialysis patients are less likely to report a pre-morbid psychiatric history than regular CL patients, they are equally likely to have a history of past substance abuse. In addition, mean scores on the Global Assessment of Functioning Scale and Hamilton Anxiety and Hamilton Depression Scales are less impaired in the dialysis patients.

3. Screening in the Kidney Transplant Process

It has been suggested that patients with anxiety and depression should be screened out of the selection process. Post-transplant depression, anxiety and insomnia have been shown to compromise QOL despite a successful kidney transplant. The correlation of quality and duration of sleep and positive mental health has become a matter of interest to psychologists formulating intervention. Twenty organ transplant recipients were enrolled in an eight-week course of stress reduction where they were instructed in relaxation techniques such as meditation and gentle *Hatha Yoga*. The intervention was followed up with homework assignments and practice diaries. Intervention was analyzed in terms of the impact on symptoms of stress, illness intrusion and transplant related stressors. The long-term impact of stress reduction in terms of duration and quality of sleep continued for six months after completion of treatment, as did self-report measures of anxiety and depression.

Patients who experience psychological problems during dialysis have long been considered high risk for kidney transplant. The reasoning behind such thinking has largely been based on the assumption that a relationship exists between emotional stability and non-adherence with the post-transplant regime and potential psychopharmacological interactions between psychotropic and immunosuppressive medications.

4. Effect of Modifying Immunosuppressive Therapy

The side-effects of immunosuppressant medication, the most distressing being pain, weakness, weight gain and facial changes and subsequent negative effects on QOL in patients who receive a successful transplant have been addressed using Mindfulness-Based Stress Reduction (MBSR) over a course of eight weeks. The authors reported significant improvement from baseline symptom scores for depression and insomnia. However, the authors pointed to the non-controlled social support effect of the treatment that they observed benefited the patients, such as group support and attention of the instructor. The challenge has been to determine the aspects of immunosuppressive medication that act as modifiers and those that have an adverse effect on patient wellbeing. One hundred and fifty seven kidney transplants patients from two transplant centers, with a graft that had been functioning for a minimum of seven years, were subjected to a stress based interview concerning the adverse side-effects of their immunosuppressive medication as well as their past level of educational achievement and available social support. In addition, a socio-medical profile was compiled for each patient from medical records concerning type of dialysis intervention, immunosuppressant protocols, type of organ received and length of time after transplant. The findings suggested that the most stressful symptoms were pain, weakness, weight gain, facial changes, depression and anxiety and thought, in part, to correlate to the trend in continued unemployment post-transplant. Women and patients of low educational achievement were more likely to suffer from the adverse effects of immunosuppressive medication. However, age, social support, dialysis modality before transplant, time from transplant and type of immunosuppressive treatment did not impact upon individual patient score regarding stress from adverse effects. Adverse effects of immunosuppressants can also impact upon morbidity and mortality. Negative effects of immunosuppressants concerning appearance, mood and energy can impact upon patient's mood more than metabolic changes due to their ability to impact upon the morale and emotional well-being of patients. The authors concluded overall, that despite their side- effects, immunosuppresant medications can lead to improved QOL, decrease non-adherence and prevent graft loss.

However, the controlled withdrawal of immunosuppressants has also been equated with the onset of anxiety (Sanfey 1997). Steroid withdrawal was offered to a group of twenty-five male and eighteen female patients who had a stable, functioning graft for at least one year with only mild episodes of rejection. Maintenance immunosuppression in all patients consisted of CSA 3-5mg/kg and AZA 1-2mg/kg. Twenty-nine patients (67 percent) have remained off steroids with good renal function for 13-59 months. The authors concluded that patients who had experienced episodes of anxiety were not good candidates for withdrawal of immunosuppressants.

5. Group Therapy

Group therapy for dialysis and transplant patients has consistently been demonstrated to be an effective forum for the treatment of these patients (Baines 2004). Authors have pointed to the opportunity to observe other group members and learn from their coping and adaptive strategies.

6. Kidney Transplant as a Panacea for Dialysis Anxiety

There appears to be a common expectation that transplant is an instant panacea for dialysis anxiety, which is not wholly supported by the data. In a cohort study ninety-seven transplant patients were screened pre-transplant and two weeks post-transplant using the General Health Questionnaire (CHQ-28) and the Minnesota Multiphasic Personality Inventory (MMPI) (Arapslan 2004). The results suggested that CHQ-28 rates showed significant improvement two weeks post-transplant. Patients who had a pre-morbid psychiatric history prior to transplant were significantly less likely to demonstrate change in CHQ-28 scores. The findings suggested that the patients who received a cadaver kidney transplant were more liable to become anxious and depressed than their living kidney recipients. The findings were further correlated in terms of the cadaver kidney recipients having to contend with both the uncertainty as to when, if ever, they will receive a timely transplant, along with the waiting time for surgery. Also, when relatives failed to come forward as donors, patients often harbored feelings of rejection. Studies that have compared anxiety and depression in patients who receive living as opposed to cadaver transplants have suggested that there were no long term significant difference in terms of depression and anxiety, although 20 percent all of patients were found to be suffering from depression irrespective of whether or not they received a living or cadaver transplant (Schlebusch 1989). Depression and anxiety in the cadaver kidney transplant recipients was linked to concerns about the psychological and personal characteristics of the donor.

Some studies that have suggested that while dialysis patients may be more depressed than transplant patients, transplant patients are more likely to be suffering from anxiety (Teran-Escandon 2001). The transplant process can be very anxiety provoking, irrespective of whether the patient is waiting for a living kidney or cadaver kidney donor. Waiting time for surgery and the availability of a donor have been found to be the main precipitating factors.

Conclusion

The need for a better understanding of the emotional aspects of dialysis and organ transplant and the case for psychological intervention have been made repeatedly in publications and books dealing with dialysis and transplantation. It has been suggested that the emotional presentation of dialysis and organ transplant patients is much more complex than originally thought and that intervention has been fragmented and intermittent. Further, that failure to recognize and intervene amongst these patients can lead to graft loss and even death.

Chapter 11:
Social Networks in Kidney Transplantation

In contrast to the early studies that placed emphasis upon the donor, contemporary studies amongst live related and unrelated transplants have placed emphasis upon the donor and recipient as an interactive pair[54]. In addition, we suggest that the donor and recipient relationship needs to be analyzed within the context of any external points of influence such as social networks in which the donor or recipient may be embedded. The psychosocial history or background of individuals presenting for transplant is undoubtedly intertwined with the medical outcome of the transplant. Renal disease and transplantation plays out within the context of family attitudes, values, beliefs, culture, and the relational history of the family. Rather like the geneticist who gathers patient and family history as a means to determine pre-disposition to illness, we profile our patients and their social networks to determine what aspects might predispose, or compromise them relationally after a successful transplant.

We place emphasis upon understanding the relational history of donors and recipients, as a means to act as a template, and precursor to effective supportive intervention and the making of an informed decision about surgery. We prefer to invite potential live donors and their recipients to attend at least three preparatory sessions prior to transplant. Within the context of the sessions, psychotherapy is seen as a vehicle of insight and change before surgery. In this chapter, we have discussed the characteristics of relationships, interaction and

---

54   Sajjad I, Baines LS, Salifu M, Jindal RM. The dynamics of recipient-donor relationships in living kidney transplantation. American Journal of Kidney Diseases 2007; 50:834

communication patterns that we observe in our patients during these sessions.

There is also the matter of individual change, or transition that affects all of our lives and that accompanies personal development. A thread running throughout this book is the curtailment of lifestyle and a pervasive sense of powerless synonymous with low mood that most renal patients, either side of transplant, experience at some point. We have also seen how post-transplant patients move through a period of personal transition. People do not implement change in their lives apart from their personal relationships. Therefore, the donor-recipient relationship will need to be one that has withstood change in the past or that might be open to change in the future. Psychotherapy can often be a vehicle for change.

Many of the instruments that measure or attempt to understand personal relationships do so from an idealist perspective. This might include evenly balanced (power and support) relationships with kin, a varied supportive social network, a firm sense of personal identity, a track record of enduring intimacy and romantic attachments, personal development, ability to effectively communicate feelings and emotions, along with the ability to effectively manage conflict and disappointment and the ending of these relationships. Variations on these scenarios are often seen as a deviation and may count against the donor or recipient.

The key to gaining insight into the nature of a patient's relationship patterns in the present, along with their ability to form and retain attachments lies in their past. That is, the nature and characteristics of early attachments (usually with primary care givers) are direct determinants of adult personality and emotional wellbeing. Also the way in which individuals interact and behave in relationships are a direct reflection of their past experience of being in relationships.

However, amongst renal or any other patient who has lived with a chronic illness the presentation is slightly more complex. We have seen throughout the book that renal disease, dialysis, and transplantation can have a negative effect upon personal relationships and development. This renders patients to become quite isolated, dependent upon a small number of family and friends, often with fluctuating mood and low self-esteem. Therefore, any pre-transplant evaluation would need to reflect the experience of living with an uncertain prognosis. As seen earlier, concerning compliance issues, we place emphasis on understanding the relational history of the donor and the recipient, as a means to act as a template and to increase insight and institute supportive intervention. This generally takes the form of addressing any old hostilities or misunderstandings. The psychotherapist will need to be willing to challenge any mismatches or imbalance in the relationship while reinforcing supportive qualities. This leads to an informed decision on the part of the donor and recipient. We have provided below a brief overview below of the characteristics of relationships that we sensitize ourselves over 3-4 sessions of therapy in preparation for living kidney transplant.

Characteristics of Relationships in Live Kidney Transplants

Donor-Recipient Relationship: A mutually acceptable pattern of attachment entails complementary thought processes, interpersonal behavior and corresponding mood. Within the context of the donor-recipient relationship, the therapist would need to identify episodes of interaction with attention to whether both parties felt understood by the other and the appropriateness of the time frame and manner of the response. We also need to understand the nature of the response, counter-responses from the other party, counter-responses and implications for other social network members.

Characterization of Donor-Recipient Behavior: A mutually satisfactory relationship is thought to be in keeping with the life style, attitudes, values and beliefs of the parties involved. Therefore, within the context of the donor-recipient relationship we would be concerned to observe inflexibility, extreme attitudes, values and beliefs that appear to oppose, or be hostile to those of the other party. There are three main behavior scenarios that are liable to misinterpretation and therefore we should be alert are as follows:

Avoiding-disengaging behavior: Is associated with avoidance of commitment and usually manifests as feelings of vulnerability and fear of rejection. These individuals have a personal sense of insecurity, a tendency to distrust others and avoid close relationships. This behavior is usually symptomatic of such feelings towards a specific individual, or as a result of growing up in a family where expression of emotion and intimacy was not encouraged. This is most easily identified when meeting with donor families in terms of social roles and individuals being stereotyped, as either one thing or another, e.g. good or bad, clever or stupid. These patients have often forgotten or cannot recollect whole portions of their childhood. This type of behavior is inherent and has usually been passed down through the generations and is very difficult to change. They are unlikely to come forward as donors or as recipients as they would have difficulty accepting an organ.

Ambivalent-enmeshed behavior: These individuals are liable to apply emotional pressure on others to gain attention and prompt others to respond to their needs; become over dependent on others and will often idealize them. They are usually identifiable by virtue of their tendency to carry a great deal of unresolved emotional baggage from the past. Their tactics of keeping past disagreements alive and attributing deceased family member's personas to current family members also has the effect of confusing and dispersing the rest of their social network. They will have a tendency to present with long convoluted stories and will have high expectations of other social network members, who will often try to avoid them. As potential recipients they will have high expectations that family members will donate to them. However, as donors they may offer to donate, but will be illusive and their offer will never quite materialize.

Transitions: This is the manner in which changes in roles, settings, endings or beginnings have been managed in the past. Such periods of time are quite emotive as they often render the individual quite vulnerable to anxiety. However, they often also offer the opportunity for personal development particularly transitions in health status after the transplant. Relationships are not static but are dynamic and can be activated by relational, social or environmental circumstances. Therefore, the donor-recipient relationship will need to be one that has withstood change in the past, or that might be open to change in the future.

Social Support for Live Kidney Transplantation: A number of health studies have placed a significant amount of emphasis upon the extent of social support afforded to patients; both as an indicator of their ability to endure some form of treatment intervention and as a means to generate security and confidence. However, less attention is given to the fact that social support can cause stress as well as allay it. It is not wise therefore, to assume that a patient has sufficient social support just because he or she is married as an example. Social support can also be conditional, upon the other behavior, attitudes, values or beliefs remaining constant, or in keeping with that of the supporter. There may be occasions when another member of the social network needs support as well due to the onset of an illness. This can serve to destabilize or unbalance the network by being viewed as competition or neglect by other members. Subsequent attention seeking behavior by patients on dialysis or transplant could seriously unbalance the network.

Individual Differences: Individual difference, or an individual's conscious concept of their thoughts and feelings, both in relationship to themselves and others, has been referred to directly and indirectly throughout the book. Within the context of the donor-recipient relationship, there needs to be some measure and acceptance of individual difference, peculiarities and idiosyncrasies. A family or peer social network that is able to accommodate individual difference without ridicule or exclusion, will have demonstrated that it is flexible and tolerant.

Conflict: Individual differences may well be associated with conflict. However, the existence of conflict within the donor-recipient relationship does not in itself pose an obstacle to live transplantation. However, the therapist will need to be alert to whether the conflict appears constructive or destructive. Constructive conflict is associated with either ongoing or newly acquired insight, attitudes or values that are synonymous with relational growth and mutual satisfaction. However, destructive conflict tends to stagnate a relationship and leaves one or both parties unsatisfied. Destructive conflict is often associated with poor and/or inappropriate communication skills, which in turn, is usually associated with differing, but not necessarily irreconcilable perspectives of a problem.

Disparity In Shared Family Experience: It is quite common to encounter two siblings from the same family who have completely incongruent memories of a parent or another sibling. Listening to these patients it is almost as though they grew up in different families. There are generally two reasons for this, firstly, that the experience of the parent on the part of the child is determined by the life stage or events that are ongoing in the parent's life when they are born into the family. Secondly, a child by coincidence of the timing of his or her birth becomes representative of a time point in the parent's relationship, or coincides with the death of a significant family member. In the latter instance, the child's own personality traits can be suppressed in order for him or her to be attributed the characteristics of the lost family member. This scenario can of course manifest in both a favorable or unfavorable manner. In adulthood, such experiences can result in covert resentment, or feelings of being indebted to other family members.

PART III

Chapter 12:

Economics of Kidney Transplantation in Developing Countries

Incidence of kidney failure: The number of patients requiring renal replacement therapy either by dialysis or kidney transplantation is estimated to be about 1.4 million and is growing at the rate of 8 percent annually[55]. A number of factors may account for this increase: diabetes, ageing population and hypertension are the major factors. It may be difficult to estimate the burden of renal failure in developing countries, as there is a lack of national registries with some notable exception. However, it is anticipated that the incidence of kidney failure is likely to increase due to a dramatic rise in the incidence of diabetic nephropathy. Developing countries also have a high incidence of infectious causes of kidney disease. The role of environmental pollution and herbal medicines in causing kidney failure is still being explored[56].

The population of Guyana is estimated to be 751,223[57] by the most recent resent estimates. Because of similarities in ethnic composition and socio-economic conditions, it would be ideal to extrapolate the incidence of patients requiring renal replacement therapy from India, however, there is no national registry in India and the incidence of renal replacement therapy in India may be under-reported. Therefore,

---

55   Schieppati A, Remuzzi G. Chronic renal disease as a public health problem: epidemiology, social, and economic implications. Kidney Int Suppl 2005; 68:7-10.

56   White SL, Chadban SJ, Jan S, Chapman JR, Cass A. How can we achieve global equity in provision of renal replacement therapy?

57   http://schools-wikipedia.org/wp/g/Guyana.htm

it may not be unreasonable to use the data from Singapore; where the incidence of new end-stage renal failure treated with dialysis was ninety-six per million in 1992 and is 167 per million in 2000. It would, therefore be reasonable to assume that approximately 200 new patients per year would need renal replacement therapy in Guyana. As there is no national registry for this in Guyana and only one hemodialysis center, it could be assumed that most patients are either dying of renal failure or receiving dialysis or transplantation outside the country. The increase in the incidence of diabetes and hypertension throughout the developing world would mean that the number of patients requiring renal replacement therapy is likely to increase considerably.

The incidence of renal failure varies from country to country, some of the differences could be due to lack of national registries, under-reporting, and large people may die from kidney failure without receiving renal replacement therapy (RRT) in the form of dialysis or kidney transplantation. The incidence of new end-stage renal disease (ESRD) treated with dialysis in Singapore has risen from ninety-six per million population (pmp) in 1992 to 167 pmp in 2000. This near-doubling is not unique to Singapore, and many other Asian countries have seen a similar increase in the incidence of end stage renal failure, in large part due to an increasing incidence of the risk factors for renal disease. Consequent to this high incidence of renal failure, at the end of 2002, an estimated 301,649 patients were on dialysis in Asia[58].

There is an epidemiological transition taking place in India, with the decline in communicable diseases and a growing burden of chronic disease: a situation perhaps similar in Guyana. In a recent review, Reddy and others noted that 53 percent of deaths in India in 2005 were due to chronic disease. The principal named categories of chronic disease in their report were cardiovascular disease, cancer, chronic respiratory disease and diabetes. Notably, chronic kidney disease (CKD) was not a category on 'its' own merits but most likely included under the 'other' category[59]. The World Health Organization laid down certain criteria for a major non-communicable disease (NCD), namely, (i) being a major cause of morbidity and mortality, (ii) being amenable to prevention by community-based strategies, and (iii) sharing common

---

58   http://annals.edu.sg/pdf200502/edit341.pdf
59   Rao M, Pereira BJG. Chronic kidney disease in India – a hidden epidemic. In J Med Res

risk factors with other NCDs. Though CKD meets these criteria, it does not find a place in this category. There is no reason to suspect that the global epidemic of CKD does not have its counterpart in India and epidemiologic indicators suggest that it is likely to be sizeable.

Cost effectiveness of dialysis versus kidney transplantation: There is a vast body of literature that has shown that kidney transplantation is more cost effective than dialysis, both in terms of lower cost and improved quality of life. In developing countries this is particularly important as dialysis facilities may be non-existence or too expensive. Even taking into account the cost of immunosuppressants, kidney transplant is more cost effective. In fact, utility values for dialysis were 0.65 for the first six months of dialysis and 0.68 after the first six months[60]. On the other hand, the utility value for transplantation was 0.84. This should not deter from preventative measures to reduce kidney disease.

Survival advantage of kidney transplantation: Studies have clearly shown that a successful kidney transplant will improve patient survival compared to patient remaining on dialysis. Investigators assessed the magnitude of the survival benefit of renal transplantation compared with dialysis in Scotland[61]. In a longitudinal study of survival and mortality risk in 1732 adult patients, the relative risk (RR) of death during the first 30 days after transplantation was 1.35 compared with patients on dialysis (RR = 1). The long-term RR (at 18 mo) for the transplant recipients was 0.18 when compared with patients on dialysis (RR = 1). The projected life expectancy with a transplant was 17.19 yr compared with only 5.84 yr on dialysis. Wolfe et al.[62] conducted a longitudinal study of mortality in 228,552 patients who were receiving long-term dialysis for end-stage renal disease. Of these patients, 46,164 were placed on a waiting list for transplantation, 23,275 of whom received a first cadaveric transplant between 1991 and 1997. Among the various subgroups, the

---

60 Hornberger JC, Best JH, Garrison Jr LP. Cost-effectiveness of repeat medical procedures: kidney transplantation as an example. Med Decis Making 1997; 17: 363-72.

61 Oniscu GC, Brown H, Forsythe JL. Impact of cadaveric renal transplantation on survival in patients listed for transplantation. J Am Soc Nephrol 2005;16:1859.

62 Wolf RA, et al. Comparison of mortality in all patients on dialysis, patients on dialysis awaiting transplantation, and recipients of a first cadaveric transplant. N Engl J Med 1999; 341:1725.

standardized mortality ratio for the patients on dialysis who were awaiting transplantation (annual death rate, 6.3 per one hundred patient-years) was 38 to 58 percent lower than that for all patients on dialysis (annual death rate, 16.1 per one hundred patient-years). The relative risk of death during the first two weeks after transplantation was 2.8 times as high as that for patients on dialysis who had equal lengths of follow-up since placement on the waiting list, but at eighteen months the risk was much lower (relative risk, 0.32; 95 percent confidence interval, 0.30 to 0.35; P<0.001). The likelihood of survival became equal in the two groups within five to 673 days after transplantation in all the subgroups of patients we examined. The long-term mortality rate was 48 to 82 percent lower among transplant recipients (annual death rate, 3.8 per one hundred patient-years) than patients on the waiting list, with relatively larger benefits among patients who were twenty to thirty-nine years old, white patients, and younger patients with diabetes.

Rabbat et al. investigated if kidney transplantation offers a survival advantage in regions where dialysis survival is superior to that in the United States in a cohort of 1156 patients who started end-stage renal disease therapy and were wait-listed for cadaveric renal transplantation in Ontario, Canada between January 1, 1990 and December 31, 1994. Patients were followed from wait listing for renal transplant (n = 1156), to cadaveric first renal transplant (n = 722), to death, or to study end. The average RR of dying was 2.91 in the first thirty days after transplantation, but was significantly lower one year after transplantation, indicating a beneficial long-term effect when compared to wait listed dialysis patients[63].

Survival benefit was observed even with Expanded Criteria Donor (ECD) kidney transplants. In a retrospective cohort study using data from a US national registry of mortality and graft outcomes among kidney transplant candidates and recipients; ECD recipients had a 27 percent lower risk of death. However, in areas with shorter waiting times, only recipients with diabetes demonstrated an ECD survival benefit[64].

63   Rabbat CG, Thorpe KE, Russell JD, Churchill DN. Comparison of mortality risk for dialysis patients and cadaveric first renal transplant recipients in Ontario, Canada. J Am Soc Nephrol 2000;11:917.

64   Merion RM, Ashby VB, Wolfe RA, et al. Deceased-donor characteristics and the survival benefit of kidney transplantation. JAMA 2005;294:2726.

Cost of dialysis in Guyana: In the context of Guyana, the cost of dialysis at the country's only dialysis unit is as below:
http://5gdialysis.com/about.html 5G, Guyana's first hemodialysis center, was established in order to satisfy the unmet need for dialysis in Guyana. Operational since July 2005. The cost per treatment for long-term patients is US$175, and for transient (visiting) patients is between US$200 and US$300.

Comparative costs of hemodialysis for one year are US$5000 in India, $6240 in Indonesia and $7500 in China and $7332 in Brazil. It seems that the cost of hemodialysis in Guyana is higher than in comparative countries, making it more imperative to develop a kidney transplant program[65].

Need for kidney transplants: In India, less than 10 percent of all patients receive any kind of renal replacement therapy; most patients started on hemodialysis with only a small proportion (<0.5 percent) started on continuous ambulatory peritoneal dialysis. About 60 percent are lost to follow up within three months, primarily due to economic reasons. Further in India, although renal transplantation is a cheaper option due to reduced maintenance costs over time, only about 5-10 percent of patients with kidney failure have a transplant[66]. From the various newspaper reports of people looking for help to travel abroad for kidney transplants, it would seem that a similar situation exists in Guyana where probably only 10 percent of patients receive any type of renal replacement therapy and only 5-10 percent of these receive a kidney transplant.

Burden of Chronic Kidney Disease (CKD): What then is the burden of CKD in Guyana? There is a dearth of statistics from Guyana; however, it may be of interest to study the situation in India where a comparative situation may exist. Recent publications have dealt with mainly single center reports or regional population based estimates and the definition of CKD has differed. In the absence of nationwide reporting systems or registries, the true incidence and prevalence is difficult to determine. Observational and anecdotal data suggest

65   Sakuja V, Sud K. End-stage renal disease in India and Pakistan: Burden of disease and management issues. Kidney Int (Suppl) 2003;63:115-8.

66   Sakhuja V, Kohli HS. End-stage renal disease in India and Pakistan: incidence, causes, and management. Ethn Dis 2006; 16 (2 Suppl 2) : S2-20-3

that the normal ranges of glomerular filtration rate (GFR) may be lower in the predominantly vegetarian, less muscular Indian subjects with different creatinine generation rates, compared to their western counterparts although this issue needs more rigorous study. In the last decade, there has been a major evolution in the definition and classification of CKD that is based upon estimated GFR. Application of these definitions would impact identification of disease. Therefore issues of global implementation will need to be resolved. Mani, working in Chennai, South India, estimated a prevalence of chronic renal failure of 0.16 percent in the community in 2003; applying the Modification in Diet in Renal Disease (MDRD) equation for GFR estimation in 2005, 0.86 percent was found to have a GFR 1.8 mg/dL. Estimates for the United States population extrapolated from the National Health and Nutrition Examination Survey (NHANES III) data place the prevalence of CKD stages four and five (severe decrease in GFR) and CKD stage three (moderate decrease in GFR) at 0.4 percent. However, such direct comparisons with Western populations are not valid since the equivalent GFR for a serum creatinine of 1.8 mg/dL in Indians may place the individual anywhere between CKD stages two to four depending upon gender and nutritional status.

Modi and Jha[67] reported from an urban population in the city of Bhopal, India, that the crude and age adjusted incidence rates of ESRD were 151 and 232 per million population respectively. ESRD incidence rates lend themselves more easily to international comparisons, as the diagnosis is less susceptible to inaccuracies. These estimates are roughly similar to the US. Moreover, the socioeconomic implications of a young population afflicted with a potentially terminal illness is devastating and in the face of growing epidemics of diabetes and hypertension, the burden of CKD is not likely to ease.

---

67 Modi GK, Jha V. The incidence of end-stage renal disease in India: a population-based study. Kidney Int 2006; 70(12):2131.a

Chapter 13:
Economics of Peritoneal Dialysis (PD) Versus Hemodialysis (HD)

Pertinent to this chapter is the feasibility of providing renal replacement therapy in developing countries where the issues of infectious diseases and infrastructure issues are a major problem. Renal failure affects a relatively small proportion of population, so it could be argued that the government with limited resources cannot provide free renal replacement therapy. Twenty million Americans suffer from chronic kidney disease (CKD), and twenty million more are at elevated risk; soon, one in nine Americans will have CKD. Control of co-morbidities may slow its progression, and two are critical—type 2 diabetes and hypertension[68]. The employers are only now beginning to understand the effect of this on their financing systems.

A key factor influencing the cost of dialysis care is the timing of referral to a Nephrologist[69]. When patients are either referred late to a Nephrologist's care or must urgently initiate dialysis without a planned access, they are generally sicker, require longer hospitalization and are nearly always started on HD. Early referral and planned start result in cost savings and improved survival. Patients who are referred earlier to a Nephrologist have an extended time prior to starting dialysis during which access may be planned and placed, and patients may be objectively educated about their treatment choices. This approach has usually been found to result in fewer inpatient hospital days, thereby

---

68   Sullivan S. Employer challenges with the chronic kidney disease
      population. J Manag Care Pharm 2007; 13(9 Suppl D): S19.

69   Wavamunno MD, Harris DC. The need for early nephrology referral.
      Kidney Int Suppl 2005;94: S128.

reducing the total cost of dialysis by the creation of vascular access or PD and taking steps to improve nutrition and treating infectious problems.

Horl et al. compared access to End Stage Renal Disease (ESRD) treatment modalities was made with reference to the healthcare provider structure in a range of industrial countries[70]. The countries were grouped into 'public' (Beveridge model), 'mixed' (Bismarck model) and 'private' (Private Insurance model). In 'public' provider countries, 20-52 percent of dialysis patients are treated with home therapies (haemodialysis and peritoneal dialysis), and the number of patients with renal transplants is 45-81percent of all ESRD patients. In 'mixed' provider countries, only 9-17 percent of all dialysis patients are treated with home therapies, and 20-48 percent of ESRD patients have renal transplants. In 'private' provider countries, 17 percent of the United States, and 6 percent of the Japanese dialysis patients are treated with home therapies. Japan has 0.3 percent and the United States has 26 percent of ESRD patients who receive renal transplants. It thus seems that provider structure influences access to and choice of ESRD treatment.

For Guyana to develop a renal replacement therapy as a national program, it would have to allocate resources for dialysis therapy and decide the preferred modality, HD versus PD. Should Guyana be influenced by the experience in the United States or other developing countries? Compared with countries worldwide, the United States has one of the lowest PD populations as compared with its HD population. Approximately 12 percent of the total dialysis population in the United State is on PD[71]. There have been arguments for and against each modality of therapy in the context of a developing country, but the preponderance of evidence is in favor of PD in developing countries. In a seminal paper, Just et al[72] made an argument for providing PD,

70 Horl WH, de Alvaro F, Williams PF. Healthcare systems and end-stage renal disease (ESRD) therapies--an international review: access to ESRD treatments. Nephrol Dial Transplant. 1999; 14 [Suppl 6]:10-5.

71 Gadallah MF, Ramdeen G, Torres-Rivera C, et al. Changing the trend: a prospective study on factors contributing to the growth rate of peritoneal dialysis programs. Adv Perit Dial 2001; 17:122-6.

72 Just PM, de Charro FT, Tschosik EA, Noe LL, Bhattacharyya SK, Riella MC. Reimbursement and economic factors influencing dialysis modality choice around the world. Nephrol Dial Transplant 2008; 23:2365-73.

which may be more cost effective. The costs of dialysis around the world can vary widely according to many local market conditions, including local production and distribution factors, import duties, the presence or absence of local suppliers and purchasing power. HD cost is driven largely by the fixed costs of facility space and staff. HD machines typically cost ~$18,000 to $30,000 each, but the machines have a five to ten year life cycle, and, in a weekly schedule, three to six patients can be treated on one machine. The cost of dialyzers for HD ranges from $1,000 to $5,000 per year. Other items that factor into the cost of HD are additional facility costs such as maintenance and utilities, and the costs of transportation to and from the HD facility. They further argue that the economics of PD are driven primarily by variable, or 'disposable' costs, such as the costs of solutions and dialysis tubing, and PD exhibits a near constant economy of scale. A review of the literature determined that the cost of PD materials ranges from $5,000 to $25,000 annually. The use of automated cyclers generally adds to the cost of PD. The machines cost $3,000 to $10,000 each when purchased outright. However, they may be leased or provided, in which case their actual cost is bundled into the cost of solutions and materials purchased through the same company.

A North American literature review concluded that PD is less expensive than HD and that the difference in cost is dramatic when the PD program is relatively large and well run. Lee et al. reported their cost analysis for care for in-center, satellite, and home/self-care HD and PD were US $51,252, $47,680, $42,057, $29,961, and $26,959, respectively (P < 0.001). After adjustment for the effect of other important predictors of cost, such as co-morbidity, these differences persisted. They suggested that dialysis programs should encourage the use of home/self-care HD and PD[73]. In general, reports from Western Europe are in agreement with the North American findings. A review of the literature found that in-centre HD was about twice the cost of PD in France and 30 percent more expensive than PD in Italy and the United Kingdom. The majority of the countries in South Asia lack government healthcare system for reimbursing renal replacement therapy. The largest utilization of chronic PD is in India, with nearly

73 Lee H, Manns B, Taub K, Ghali WA, Dean S, Johnson D, Donaldson C. Cost analysis of ongoing care of patients with end-stage renal disease: the impact of dialysis modality and dialysis access. Am J Kidney Dis 2002; 40:611.

6500 patients on this treatment by the end of 2006. A large majority of patients are doing two L exchanges three times per day, using glucose-based dialysis solution manufactured in India[74]. A recent conference of academic Nephrologists and government officials from China, Hong Kong, India, Indonesia, Japan, Macau, Malaysia, Philippines, Singapore, Taiwan, Thailand, and Vietnam proposed the "peritoneal dialysis first" policy model, incentive programs, nongovernmental organizations providing PD, and PD reimbursement in a developing economy[75].

Very little research exists on the economics of dialysis in developed Asian countries[76]. A multi-national survey of Asian Nephrologistss conducted in 2001 suggests that HD is generally more expensive than PD in the developed Asian economies of Hong Kong, Singapore, Taiwan and Japan. However, the extent of cost savings with PD varies by region. According to the survey results, the ratio of costs for HD compared to PD ranged from a low of 0.99-1.09 in Japan to a high of 1.42-2.39 in Hong Kong. The economics of dialysis in the developing world differ from advanced nations. PD requires less technology than HD, so it would seem particularly well suited for developing nations. In poorer countries, though, labor is relatively inexpensive, while the cost of imported equipment and solutions is high. Costs are often considered as related only to supplies rather than assessed as a total therapy. Therefore, there is often a perception that PD is more expensive than HD in developing countries. To reduce costs, patients may be placed on outdated straight-line systems and sometimes transfer sets may be reused. However, high peritonitis rates increase the cost of PD treatment even further, and dropout rates are high.

Vikrant et al[77] review their experience of PD in the Indian context and may be applicable to Guyana. They investigated the feasibility of

74 Abraham G, Pratap B, Sankarasubbaiyan S, et al. Chronic peritoneal dialysis in South Asia - challenges and future. Perit Dial Int 2008; 28:13.

75 Li PK, Lui SL, Leung CB, et al. Increased utilization of peritoneal dialysis to cope with mounting demand for renal replacement therapy--perspectives from Asian countries. Perit Dial Int 2007; 27 Suppl 2: S59.

76 Li PK, Chow KM. The cost barrier to peritoneal dialysis in the developing world--an Asian perspective. Perit Dial Int 2001; 21 [Suppl 3]: S307.

77 Vikrant S. Continuous ambulatory peritoneal dialysis: A viable modality of renal replacement therapy in a hilly state of India.

PD in hilly, remote state of India with predominant rural population with a population of 6 million involved 25 patients who were initiated on PD between October 2002 and December 2006 and who survived and/or had more than 6 months follow up on this treatment with last follow up till June 30, 2007. The total duration on PD treatment was 541.1 patient-months with a mean duration of 21.6 ± 12.2 months and median duration of nineteen patient-months (range: 6-56.3 patient-months). No patient had exit-site infection. There were twenty-six episodes of peritonitis. The rate of peritonitis was one episode per twenty-one patient-months or 0.6 per patient-year during the treatment period. The main cause of death was cardiovascular complications. Patient and technique survival at one, two, and three years was 80, 36 and 12 percent, respectively. They concluded that PD was a safe and viable mode of renal replacement in remote and rural places.

In a study by Neil et al[78] the relative advantages of HD and PD was discussed to estimate the country specific, five year financial implications on total dialysis costs assuming utilization shifts from HD to PD in two high-income (United Kingdom, Singapore), three upper-middle-income (Mexico, Chile, Romania), and three lower-middle-income (Thailand, China, Colombia) countries. They found that PD was a clinically effective dialysis option that can be significantly cost saving compared to HD, even in developing countries.

In developing countries, infections are the leading causes of morbidity and the second commonest cause of mortality in the dialysis population. Tuberculosis is endemic in several developing countries and impaired cell-mediated immunity increases the susceptibility among the dialysis population. The reported incidence of tuberculosis in dialysis patients varies from 10 to 15 percent in India. Further, the infection rate is higher in government-funded hospitals that cater to patients from the lower socioeconomic groups. The principal causes of death are cardiovascular (40-51 percent) and infections (15-23 percent).

Indian J Nephrol 2007;17:165 http://www.indianjnephrol.org/text.asp?2007/17/4/165/39171

78   Neil N, Walker DR, Sesso R, et al. Gaining Efficiencies: Resources and Demand for Dialysis around the Globe. Value Health. 2008

Chapter 14:
Pre-Emptive Kidney Transplant for Developing Countries

It has been shown that pre-emptive kidney transplantation gives better outcomes world-wide, however, in developing countries, a major advantage is that this form of therapy may be a cost-effective option, offering additional benefits to conventional transplantation. However, providing treatment for renal failure is particularly difficult in the developing countries where national incomes are not sufficient to cover even the basic requirements of their citizens[79]. Although some developing countries are making active efforts to establish cadaver (deceased) donor transplant programs, these are virtually nonexistent in the majority at this time[80]. The abject poverty in the developing world and the increasing success rate of transplantation following the discovery of cyclosporine have led to the commercialization and sale of kidneys for transplantation, an unethical practice which must be curbed, a topic we have discussed extensively in our book[81]. There is a near unanimity of opinion that renal transplantation is far cheaper than prolonged dialysis, and the benefit to the recipient is enormous in terms of the years of life saved and the quality of life.

---

79 Jha V. End-stage renal care in developing countries: the India experience. Ren Fail 2004; 26:201.

80 Chugh KS, Jha V, Chugh S. Economics of dialysis and renal transplantation in the developing world. Transplant Proc 1999; 31:3275.

81 Evans RW, Kitzmann DJ. An economic analysis of kidney transplantation. Surg Clin North Am 199; 78:149.

We believe that short periods of dialysis; either peritoneal or hemodialysis followed by transplants with living-related donor kidneys appear to be the most cost-effective treatments of renal failure.

John et al.[82] reviewed their results of forty-three patients who underwent living related pre-emptive kidney transplants versus eighty-six matched controls who underwent transplantation after hemodialysis. Controls received more transfusions, had higher hepatitis B surface antigen and more commonly had hepatic dysfunction in the pre-transplant period compared with the preemptive group. Similarly, at six months after transplant, the incidence of hepatitis B surface antigen positivity (13 vs. 2) and hepatic dysfunction (18 vs. 3) were higher in the control group compared with the preemptive group. The one and two-year graft (preemptive: 82.8 percent and 77.3 percent; controls: 82 percent and 78 percent, respectively) and patient (preemptive: 92 percent and 89.5 percent; controls: 91percent and 89.5 percent, respectively) survival rates were similar. They concluded that pre-emptive kidney transplant offers comparable patient and graft survival to conventional transplantation. It eliminates the complications and inconvenience of dialysis.

Similar experience has been shown in Egypt[83.] Between 1976 and 2001, 1,279 first living-donor transplants were performed at a single center. The eighty-two patients (6.4 percent) who underwent transplant without prior dialysis were compared with 1,197 patients who had been dialyzed before transplant. Actuarial graft and patient survival at five years was comparable in both groups. The incidence of acute and chronic rejection and mortality were similar in the two groups.

In Iran, preemptive kidney transplantation was compared to pre-transplant dialysis in 300 patients who received pre-emptive kidney transplant between 1992 and 2006 from living donors. They were compared with 300 kidney recipients receiving pre-transplant dialysis for at least six months. No significant differences were noted in the gender of the recipients, age and sex of the donors, donor source, and post-transplant immunosuppressive therapy. The authors concluded

82 John AG, Rao M, Jacob CK. Pre-emptive live-related kidney transplantation. Transplantation 1998; 66:204.

83 el-Agroudy AE, Donia AF, Bakr MA, Foda MA, Ghoneim MA. Preemptive living-donor kidney transplantation: clinical course and outcome. Transplantation 2004; 77:1366.

that in Iran, pre-emptive kidney transplant eliminates hemodialysis costs and complications[84].

In developing countries such as India, treatment of renal failure is largely guided by economic considerations; only about 5 percent of ESRD patients undergo transplant surgery[85]. Although the removal of organs from brain-dead patients has been legalized, the concept of donation of organs from deceased donors has not received adequate social sanction. Only 2 percent of all transplants are performed from deceased donors. These experiences should guide Guyana professionals and others from developing countries as they embark on setting up a treatment policy for treatment of kidney failure. Most authors conclude that in the context of a developing country, pre-emptive transplant offers comparable patient and graft survival to conventional renal transplant and eliminates the complications, inconvenience and cost of dialysis.

84 Pour-Reza-Gholi F, Nafar M, Simforoosh N, Einollahi B, Basiri A, Firouzan A, Alipour Abedi B, Farhangi S. Is preemptive kidney transplantation preferred? Updated study. Urol J 2007; 4:155.

85 Singh P, Bhandari M. Renal replacement therapy options from an Indian perspective: dialysis versus transplantation. Transplant Proc 2004; 36:2013.

Chapter 15:

Developing Health Policy for Treating Renal Failure in Developing Countries

In an ideal situation, the government should provide free care to all its citizens in some sort of a national service as in the United Kingdom or Canada. This is of course a matter of much debate and controversy[86]. This is not the place to discuss the pros and cons of different systems of health care which may range from[87] insurance-based as in the United States or a National Health System (NHS) in the United Kingdom or a mixed form as in India[88], where the government will provide only the basic health care in the country side with a few tertiary centers which provide very highly specialized forms of health care. In developing countries such as India, the management of end-stage renal disease is largely guided by economic considerations. In the absence of health insurance plans, only 5-10 percent of all patients with End stage Renal Disease (ESRD) in India obtain some form of renal replacement therapy.

It is necessary to learn from the experiences of other developing countries in setting up a health policy for Guyana. Due to the

86   Moore R, Marriott N. Cost and price in the NHS: the importance of monetary value in the decision-making framework--the case of purchasing renal replacement therapy. Health Serv Manage Res 1999;12:1.

87   Lameire N, Joffe P, Wiedemann M. Healthcare systems--an international review: an overview. Nephrol Dial Transplant 1999;14 [Suppl 6]:3.

88   Bhowmik D, Pandav CS, Tiwari SC. Public health strategies to stem the tide of chronic kidney disease in India. Indian J Public Health 2008;52:224.

population mix of Guyana, where approximately half the population is of Indian descent and the other half of African descent, analyses from India and other Caribbean countries may be particularly relevant.

Experience of Jamaica: Trisolini et al.[89] from makers develop health policy for renal failure. The results of this analysis could be useful for Guyana and developing countries, where both resources and data may be limited. Their analysis included eight issues: (1) a review of currently available clinical and scientific understanding regarding ESRD; (2) a review of country-specific socioeconomic and clinical issues relevant to ESRD in Jamaica; (3) estimates of the magnitude of the need for treatment in the Jamaican population; (4) comparison of the need with available treatment capacity; (5) cost analysis related to options for expansion of treatment capacity; (6) comparison of costs to government budget resources and other potential sources of financing; (7) development of policy options; and (8) sensitivity testing of policy scenarios and trade-offs with competing priorities. They reached a conclusion that rationing available treatment capacity may be the best option, which although politically challenging. In addition, cost saving strategies such as peritoneal dialysis, pre-emptive kidney transplantation, preventative measures and public education should be undertaken. They calculated that if all renal failure patients in Jamaica were to be treated with hemodialysis, the recurrent costs could reach 68 percent of the total Ministry of Health budget, a situation which, would be unacceptable. This is interesting as Guyana has approximately 40 percent population of African descent, and these figures could be applied to Guyana. Boston, United States, collaborated with the physicians, governmental officials and health care payers in Jamaica to help decision.

Experience of India: In India, Jha[90] has succinctly summarized the state of treatment options for renal failure. The high cost of hemodialysis puts it beyond the reach of all but the very rich and maintenance hemodialysis is the exclusively preserve of private hospitals. Government-run hospitals concentrate on renal transplantation, as this is glamorous and also is the best option for a majority of patients. India

89 Trisolini M, Ashley D, Harik V, Bicknell W. Policy analysis for end-stage renal disease in Jamaica. Soc Sci Med 1999; 49:905.

90 Jha V. End-stage renal care in developing countries: the India experience. Ren Fail 2004; 26:201.

does not have state-funded or private health insurance schemes and patients have to raise finances; however this may change due to the recent introduction of employer-based health care systems. Physicians in India have empirically tried to reduce costs by cutting down the frequency of dialysis, use of cheaper cellulosic dialyzers, dialyzer reuse and non-utilization of erythropoietin. There is no organized cadaver donation program and an overwhelming majority of transplants are performed using living donors. They concluded that the financial burden of renal replacement therapy in developing nations impacts on the lifestyle and future of entire families, and extracts a cost far higher than the actual amount of money spent on treatment.

Experience of Guatemala: Of relevance may be the experience in Guatemala[91], a country in Central America, where the health issues may be similar to that in Guyana. It is estimated that only 35 percent of Guatemalan patients with end stage renal disease would be diagnosed and treated, and unlike many developed countries, the age of presentation in 60 percent of the patients is before the forth decade. Therefore, the cost of death and disability due to a chronic renal failure in this young population is particularly profound, resulting in reduced productivity and economic growth of the country. It is also estimated that 400 pediatric cases develop progressive kidney disorder (neurogenic bladder, reflux nephropathy, chronic glomerulonephritis) annually, which, if left untreated, could result in ESRD in adulthood.

Experience of Pakistan: Pakistan is fairly representative of a developing country. It has a population of 140 million, with two-thirds of the people living in rural areas. The per capita income is less than US$500 and health expenditure by the government is 0.9 percent of gross national product (GNP). Overall, 33 percent people live below the poverty line with only $1 a day for sustenance. Life expectancy is sixty-one years for males and sixty-three for females.

Rizvi et al.[92] from Sindh Institute of Urology and Transplantation (SIUT), Dow Medical College, Karachi, Pakistan, have developed a

91 Lou-Meda R. ESRD in Guatemala and a model for preventive strategies: outlook of the Guatemalan Foundation for Children with Kidney Diseases. Ren Fail 2006; 28:689.

92 Rizvi SAH, Naqvi SAA, Hussain Z, et al. Prevention and Treatment of Renal Disease. Kidney Int 2003; 63: S96.

unique community-government partnership, which has been successful over 15-18 years. They carry out 110 transplants a year, with free after care and immunosuppressive drugs. According to their estimates, in Pakistan the prevalence of ESRD is 100 pmp. For a population of 140 million there are 150 dialysis centers, mostly in the private sector where dialysis costs US$25 per session. Of the fifteen transplant-centers, ten are in the private sector where a transplant costs between US$6 to 10,000, which is exorbitant for the vast majority of the population. The "free" transplantation costs to SIUT are $1,640 for transplant surgery and $300 per month for immunosuppressive drugs. SIUT spends $1.6 million each year only on transplantation. They have consistently reported excellent results; of the more than 1000 transplants have been performed with one and five-year graft survival of 92 percent and 75 percent and one and five-year patient survival of 94 percent and 81 percent, respectively. However, the problem of post-transplant infections continues to be a major issue; with 15 percent developing tuberculosis, 30 percent cytomegalovirus, and nearly 50 percent bacterial infections.

Experience of Thailand: Prakongsai et al.[93] explored the policy options renal replacement therapy for end-stage renal disease patients under universal coverage in Thailand. They investigated various options, efficiency in utilization of government heath resources and equity in access to health care. They found that although neither hemodialysis nor peritoneal dialysis was cost-effective due to its expensive costs per life year saved, but a wider societal concern of protecting households against financial catastrophe justified public funding treatment of renal failure, and to be feasible, rationing is unavoidable. They proposed that prevention of renal failure and provision of renal replacement therapy to every patient, up to an age cut-off, or to every patient with a defined number of renal replacement years by providing more years to the younger patients. These two options were financially feasible and achieve ethical principles of providing an equal chance to all patients, while the other two alternatives which provide life-time medical services to all or select some, would become relatively less possible. However, they recommended significant improvement in health services for preventative strategies and a centralized system of purchasing key medications such as peritoneal dialysis solution and erythropoietin

93   http://papers.ssrn.com/sol3/papers.cfm?abstract_id=1072047

injection, and finally there should be a mandatory report of all ESRD patients on newly created "Thailand Registry of Renal Replacement Therapies."

Experience of Bangladesh: Rashid et al.[94] describe their experience of managing patients with renal failure and kidney transplant in their country of 128 million people, 75 percent live in rural areas and the annual per capita GNP is $380, which is less than many developing countries discussed in this book. As expected, treatment of ESRD has low priority in. As seen in other countries, including India, less than 10 percent of ESRD patients are able to maintain dialysis in private hospitals. The majority of patients present late in the course of their disease. More than 80 percent of patients presenting with ESRD are usually unaware of their disease. Therefore, most of them either dialyze by temporary access like Jugular or femoral catheterization. Peritoneal dialysis is done if hemodialysis is not available. The survival rates for the patients on three times per week dialysis schedule were 77 percent and 57 percent at three and five years, whereas those on twice per week dialysis had survival rates of 55 percent and 40 percent at three and at five years, respectively. Renal transplantation is not as expensive as dialysis and is less costly in the university hospital than in private hospitals, in particular pre-emptive kidney transplant. There is one kidney transplant center in the university hospital and another in the private sector. A total of 458 renal transplant patients were registered between 1981 and 2001. All patients usually receive cyclosporine, azathioprine and prednisolone for three to six months then cyclosporine is withdrawn within six months to one year due to financial reasons. The graft survival in their report was 90 percent and 80 percent at one and five years, respectively. The mean age of transplant patients was thirty-six years, whereas the mean donors' age is forty years. The donors included parents; especially mothers, siblings; usually sisters, spouses; mostly wives and second- degree relatives; uncles and aunts. It is not known if commercial renal transplantation is performed in Bangladesh. The annual cost of hemodialysis at private hospitals can vary between US$4000-5500 for twice weekly or thrice weekly dialysis, an exorbitant amount of money in a developing country.

---

94 http://www.sjkdt.org/text.asp?2004/15/2/185/32905

Summary

Numerous developing countries are grappling with the issue of health care funding for renal failure. In a recent review, Barsoum[95] collaborated with leading Nephrologists in ten developing countries in filling a 103-item questionnaire addressing epidemiology, etiology, and management of renal failure in their respective countries on the basis of integrating available data from different sources. Through this joint effort, it was possible to identify a number of important trends. These include the expected high prevalence of renal failure, despite the limited access to renal replacement therapy, and the dependence of prevalence on wealth. Glomerulonephritis, rather than diabetes, remains as the main cause of chronic renal disease with significant geographical variations in the prevailing histopathological types. The implementation of different modalities of renal replacement therapy was inhibited by the lack of funding, although governments, insurance companies, and donations usually constitute the major sponsors. Hemodialysis is the preferred modality in most countries with the exception of Mexico where chronic ambulatory peritoneal dialysis takes the lead. In several other countries, dialysis is available only for those on the transplant waiting list. Dialysis is associated with a high frequency of complications particularly HBV and HCV infections. Data on HIV are lacking. Aluminum intoxication remains as a major problem in a number of countries. Treatment withdrawal is common for socioeconomic reasons. Transplantation is offered to an average of 4 per million population (pmp).

A great deal more needs to be done; economic deprivation in developing countries and the meager expenditure on health care translates into poor transplantation activity, with a rate of less than 10 pmp in contrast to the developed world at 45 to 50 pmp. With an estimated world incidence of ESRD between 80 and 110 pmp, developed countries fulfill 30 to 35 percent of their needs as compared to 1 to 2 percent of the developing world.

---

95   Barsoum RS. Overview: end-stage renal disease in the developing world. Artif Organs 2002; 26:737.

Chapter 16:

Commercialization of Kidney Transplantation

Chronic renal failure is a devastating medical, social and economic problem for patients and their families. Renal replacement therapy is a low-priority area for healthcare planners in developing nations with two-tier healthcare delivery system. In India, Pakistan, and countries, which are a source of commercial donors, there is a shortage of Nephrologists and hospitals offering dialysis and transplantation. Dialysis is expensive; there are no state-funded or private health insurance schemes and patients have to raise finances for renal replacement therapy on their own. Tied with this is the demand for kidneys from patients in the Western countries where there is a long waiting list, up to ten years in some countries. This led to the practice of the sale of kidneys for transplant[96].

Recently, a meeting of various organizations was held and they made the following declaration "The Declaration of Istanbul proclaims that the poor who sell their organs are being exploited, whether by richer people within their own countries or by transplant tourists from abroad. Moreover, transplant tourists risk physical harm by unregulated and illegal transplantation. Participants in the Istanbul Summit concluded that transplant commercialism and tourism and organ trafficking should be prohibited. And they also urged their fellow transplant professionals, individually and through their organizations, to put an end to these unethical activities and foster safe, accountable practices that meet the needs of transplant recipients while protecting donors[97]."

---

96 Osterweil N. Black market kidney surgery offers no guarantees. MedPage [online]. Accessed September 27, 2007.

97 http://www.prnewswire.com/mnr/transplantationsociety/33914/

The government of India, partly due to adverse publicity and pressure from Transplant Societies Union health ministry has finalized the amendments to the Human Organ Transplant Act, 1994, seeks to broaden the pool of donors and increase the supply of organs by widening the definition of 'near relatives' by providing swapping of organs among needy families as well as by simplifying the procedures for cadaver transplants[98]. Only in January 1995, did the kidney scandal come to the surface through a series of incidents which, received wide media coverage and prompted public outrage causing the Indian Congress to pass legislation banning trade in commercial kidney transplants. On January 15, 1995, Customs department in New Delhi uncovered a "kidney tour" racket in which donors were enticed to go abroad for removal and subsequent transplant of their kidneys. Hundreds of donors were believed to have gone on such kidney tours. On January 23, 1995 it was discovered that residents of a rehabilitation colony for leprosy patients near Madras, were found to freely donate kidneys for money offered by agents. Then, on January 29, 1995, police busted a massive racket in Bangalore. Prominent doctors in a leading city hospital had removed the kidneys, of nearly 1,000 unsuspecting people. The "donors" had been lured with offers of jobs and their kidneys removed under the pretext or removing blood. They also propose a ban on the donation of organs to foreigners by Indians, marking a blow to the illegal practice which saw 'Dr.' Amit Kumar amassing a fortune by lining up Indian 'donors' for his foreign clientele who, unable to source the organs back home, came to India[99].

The United Kingdom on the other hand recognizing that it may legally be impossible to prevent recipients going abroad to obtain kidney transplants has proposed system of presumed consent where patients' organs would be made available for transplant after death unless they had explicitly opted out or their families objected. However, it remains to be seen this is passed into law[100].

I have put these two news reports below, from the Caribbean region, to highlight the problems encountered in sending patients to India or other countries for kidney transplants. The first report is of

98   http://www.american.edu/TED/KIDNEY.HTM
99   http://timesofindia.indiatimes.com/India/New_transplant_policy_to_curb_rackets/articleshow/3718196.cms
100 http://www.guardian.co.uk/society/2008/nov/16/organ-donation-reforms

patients getting poor care in Pakistan and the second news report shows a successful kidney transplant received in India but at a tremendous cost to the family. There is no reason to believe that the cases listed here were done illegally, however, commercialization of kidney transplants is a growing problem.

Pakistan kidney transplants worry Trinidad [101]

Wednesday, July 7, 2004

PORT OF SPAIN, Trinidad (AFP): The deaths of three Trinidadians who received kidney transplants in Pakistan are causing local doctors to query the procedures, local press reported Tuesday.

The Trinidad and Tobago Medical Association was shocked by the practice of agents who lure Trinidadians to Pakistan for transplants, its public relations officer said.

"The practice is unethical and should never been allowed," Hari Maharaj told the Trinidad Express newspaper. He said the association was vigorously taking up the matter.

The three patients died within weeks of returning home, after paying 19,000 dollars each for the operation, according to the Express.

However, Abu Bakr Khan, who has been described as a kidney transplant coordinator based in Pakistan, told the paper that hospitals in that country were performing the operations along accepted standards.

According to the report, he made arrangements for some 30 patients from Trinidad to have such transplants at four hospitals: Massood, Mumtaz, National and Shariff.

The operation became popular because it costs a fraction of it costs in the United States and Canada.

101 http://www.caribbeannetnews.com/2004/07/07/transplants.htm

Leading urologist Lall Sawh was quoted as saying Trinidad should enact a bill that would allow harvesting of organs from cadavers in Trinidad.

Reena Sultan gets new lease on life following kidney transplant [102]

April 27, 2008, By Stabroek staff
Young wife and mother Reena Sultan who had been suffering from end-stage kidney disease says she has a new lease on life now that she has had a kidney transplant. It was paid for through the generosity of various organizations and individuals.

In an interview with Stabroek News yesterday she said the fight had not been easy but gratitude was the sentiment uppermost in her mind. Getting her life back on track and taking care of her husband and son was her goal now, although she could not tax herself too much. Reena Sultan and her husband Fazil returned to Guyana on April 12 after almost four months spent in India, where she underwent a kidney transplant at the Colombia Asia Hospital in Bangalore India.

Expressing joy at seeing their son again after four months, Fazil also jokingly conveyed his relief at not having to cook any more.

The couple said that their initial budget of US$15,000 was exceeded, since the actual cost of the surgery and spending four months in India came to about US$26,000, with rent taking up a lot of their finances. Renting one small apartment cost them US$1,000 per month. Reena's health problems started several years ago when she collapsed one morning at home. She was rushed to the Georgetown Public Hospital and was diagnosed with a "kidney problem." Reena's entire

---

102 http://www.stabroeknews.com/news/reena-sultan-gets-new-lease-on-life-following-kidney-transplant/

life changed from that day on. She was advised to join a clinic where a specific diagnosis was subsequently made: Reena had end stage renal disease – her kidneys had failed permanently.

The desperate fight to stay alive then began, and her condition deteriorated to the point where she could hardly walk and began to suffer from selective amnesia. She was dependent on dialysis treatment twice weekly which at that time cost US$200 per treatment.

Her husband at this point had quit his job to take care of her at home and had literally taken to the streets to ask for the funds for the kidney transplant Reena so desperately needed. It was hard work and many times he was met with insults and a 'don't care' attitude, but the sum was slowly and painfully accumulated and the couple, along with Reena's brother who was to donate his kidney, left for India on December 18, 2007.

There more trials awaited them.

When undergoing preliminary checks it was discovered that Reena's brother Ryan could not be the donor since he had a "leaky valve" in his heart. Her other brother Devaraymond Kissoon then had to fly to India to donate his kidney instead – an additional expense on the already strained budget.

However, after 29 dialyses the surgery was finally performed. Reena has to return to India in October for the standard check-up, but she said she was not sure if she would be able to go on account of the cost. She was hoping, she said, that God would smile down on her once again. She planned to go back to work after her six months convalescent period was up, but for now she was happy to do little things for herself, husband and child. In the meantime, she said, her in-laws were trying their best to make things easier for her.

After going through all of the difficulties the couple wishes to advise other persons who may have to venture down this path to have their preliminary checks done here to ensure their donor was healthy, since it was more expensive to have this done abroad.

The couple said that this experience had given them a new appreciation for life and each other. And they were extremely grateful for the support of all of those who had contributed to their cause. Fazil expressed his heartfelt appreciation to Mr and Mrs Gafoor, CIOG, Tony Yassin of Guyana Watch, Bish Panday of P and P Insurance and all the other organizations and individuals, who whatever the size of their donation had contributed to Reena being alive today.

There is an increasing trend for patients from the Western countries and Guyana to travel to various countries in the Eastern hemisphere for medical tourism (Chugh 1996; Davidson 1994). We recently published an extensive review of the outcomes of donors and recipients of kidney transplants to sensitize patients and their physicians about the poor outcomes[103]. Commercialization of body parts, in particular, of kidneys has been present for many years, but we believe this has increased due to increase in the waiting list for kidney transplants and better hospital amenities in the countries of the Eastern hemispheres (Bramstedt 2007; Walsh 2007). Legislation and edicts from various transplant societies have failed to prevent this practice[104].

In fact, there are several reports of a "kidney bazaar" flourishing in India, Pakistan and some other developing countries[105.] A cursory search

103 Sajjad I, Baines LS, Patel R, Salifu M, Jindal RM. Commercialization of kidney transplants: A systemic review of outcomes in recipients and donors. American Journal of Nephrology 2008; 28:744.

104 Commercialization in transplantation: the problems and some guidelines for practice. The Council of the Transplantation Society. Lancet 1985; 28: 715.

105 The Indian kidney bazaar. http://www.indiatogether.org/combatlaw/vol4/issue4/organ.htm

of the Internet using a variety of search engines revealed numerous individuals and brokers willing to sell kidneys. In India, the buying and selling of kidneys, was outlawed in 1994, but still thrives thanks to a "built-in loophole in the law"[106]. Several Indian state governments in 1995 adopted the Transplantation of Human Organs Act, 1994. This followed a well-publicized police crackdown on an organized kidney trade of alarming proportions. The Act, however, is far from water tight allowing an unrelated donor, for reasons of "affection or attachment towards the recipient," to donate his or her kidney if approved by the Authorization Committee; this clause has provided cover for hundreds of illegal cash-for-kidney deals[107].

We highlight some of the reports of patients who received a kidney transplant and returned to North America: Prasad et al. (2006) in a detailed study of 20 patients who received their kidney transplants from South Asia and Middle East reported that graft survival over 3 years was worse in the commercial renal transplant recipients. Eleven patients had serious post transplant opportunistic infection. Canales et al. (2006) described their experience of 10 patients from Minneapolis. Kidney function and graft survival were generally good after overseas kidney transplantation. Major problems included incomplete peri-operative information and a high incidence of post-transplant infections.

From the ethical point of view the outcomes in donors is poor and is a cause of concern:

Outcomes of donors in Pakistan: Naqvi et al. (2007) from Pakistan in a large study of 239 donors reported that the vast majority of the donors (88 percent) had no economic improvement in their lives and 98 percent reported deterioration in their general health status. Future vending was encouraged by 35 percent to pay off debts and freedom from bondage.

Outcomes of donors in India: Goyal et al. (2002) in a seminal study of 305 commercial kidney donors in India reported that average family income declined by one third after nephrectomy. Eighty-six percent reported deterioration in their health status. Seventy-nine percent would not recommend others to sell a kidney.

---

106 Frontline: India's national magazine http://www.hinduonnet.com/fline/
fl1425/14250640.htm
107 Understanding India's kidney bazaar. http://mutiny.in/2007/09/17/
understanding-indias-kidney-bazaar/

We should point out that poor outcomes seem to get a great deal of publicity; there are also reports of excellent outcomes in selected cases:

Good outcomes after commercialization of kidney transplants: Patient and graft survival rates between commercial and non-commercial kidney transplants were found to be comparable in a few instances. However, due to the limited number of well-controlled studies, it was difficult to predict good outcomes based on the country where the transplant took place or the immunosuppressive regimen used.

Sun et al. (2006) found no significant difference in graft survival between commercial and non-commercial renal transplant recipients. The mortality rate between the two groups was comparable at ten years. Details regarding immunosuppressive protocols used were not available. Canales et al. (2006) described their experience of ten patients from Minneapolis; 8 were transplanted in Pakistan, one each in China and Iran. Kidney function and graft survival were generally good after overseas kidney transplantation. Ghods et al. (2006) showed no significant differences in graft survival between the recipients of one HLA haplotype-matched living-related donor and recipients of paid regulated living-unrelated donor transplant. Cyclosporine, azathioprine, and prednisone were used for immunosuppression before 1996; later MMF was used instead of azathioprine. Induction therapy with anti-thymocyte globulin and rarely with IL2 receptor antibodies was reserved for high-risk cases.

Ben Hamida (2001) studied twenty patients who received renal transplant overseas; fourteen patients received their transplant in Iraq and three each in Egypt and Pakistan. Graft survival rates were comparable to those of living related transplant and better than those of cadaveric transplant in Tunisia. All patients initially received a combination of cyclosporine A (8 mg/kg per day) and steroids (1 mg/kg per day). After arrival in Tunisia, azathioprine was added to this regimen and cyclosporine decreased to 5 mg/kg per day. Morad et al. (2000) in a study of 389 patients showed that the patient and graft survival at one, three, and five years of commercial kidney transplantation was comparable to the recipients of living-related kidney transplant. There was no difference in the incidence of bacterial, fungal, or viral infections between the two groups. Most patients were on cyclosporine, azathioprine, and prednisone. In another study of fifty-six patients, Hussein et al. (1996) found acceptable rate of patient and graft survival despite early infectious and urologic complications. Seventy three percent of their patients were on triple therapy with cyclosporine, prednisone, and azathioprine while 23 percent were on cyclosporine and prednisone.

Poor outcomes after commercialization of kidney transplants: Majority of the studies showed inferior patient and graft survival rates in recipients of commercial kidney transplant. However, due to lack of details, it was not possible to evaluate the variables leading to poor outcomes.

Prasad et al. (2006) in a study of twenty patients who received their kidney transplants from South Asia and Middle East reported that graft survival over three years was worse in commercial transplant recipients. All patients at the time of arrival at their hospital were already on triple drug immunosuppressive regimen, with cyclosporine in seventeen, tacrolimus in five, MMF in fifteen, azathioprine in seven, and steroids in twenty-two. One patient received intravenous thymoglobulin and two received anti-CD25 antibodies for induction therapy. In a small study of eighteen patients who received their kidneys from Iraq, Frishberg et al. (1998) found a higher incidence of urologic problems, mainly as a result of inadequate uretero-vesical anastomosis. They all initially received a combination of cyclosporine and steroids. After arrival in Israel, azathioprine was added to this regimen to provide the standard triple immunosuppressive therapy.

A large number of commercial kidney transplants with inferior outcomes were performed in India. Ivanovski et al. (2005) in a study of sixteen patients showed that one, three, five, and ten-year graft survival was 78 percent, 50.2 percent, 33.3 percent, and 18.8 percent, respectively. In another study, they found a graft survival rate of 78.58 percent at the end of the first year and 64.3 percent the second year (1997). All patients received cyclosporine, prednisone and azathioprine or MMF. Inston et al. (2005) in a study of twenty-three patients from UK found an overall success rate only 44 percent. In an earlier study, Higgins et al. (2003) found that the survival rate was 68 percent and 92 percent in commercial and noncommercial renal transplant recipients, respectively. Induction immunosuppression was either tacrolimus or cyclosporine; two cases had IL2 receptor monoclonal antibody treatment. Mansy et al. (1996) in a study of twelve patients in 1996 found that two year graft survival rate was 70 percent versus 88 percent for non-commercial renal transplants. All patients received conventional immunosuppressive treatment with cyclosporine, azathioprine, and prednisone.

Discussion

The ongoing negative medical, socio-economic and emotional impact of renal failure upon patients and their families and the financial incentives for donors, appears to be driving the commercialization of organs for transplant [108]. However, research suggests that medical, socio-economic and emotional outcomes for both recipients and donors are poor[109]. While recipients are exposed to the risks of surgery in poorly equipped unsanitary clinics thereby increasing the risk of infection, donors are, in the main, drawn from the lower socio-economic groups from developing countries, who do not have access to follow up health care, or worse, they are carrying infectious diseases, such as TB, AIDS or hepatitis (Kandel 1991).

Despite donors being motivated by the opportunity to improve their financial status research has suggested that there is little or no economic improvement following donation (Naqvi 2007). Indeed, in some cases (86 percent of those surveyed) the average family income actually declined by as much as one-third after donation (Goyal 2002). These findings have been attributed to the deterioration in the donor's post-operative physical (lack of stamina) and emotional health status (anxiety and depression) due to difficulty gaining access to follow up health care and subsequent ability to gain paid employment (Zargooshi 2001).

The reported deterioration in physical stamina could be linked to the emotional issues of depression and anxiety. However, further studies have suggested that despite motivations for donation being financial; the negative behavior and apparent lack of gratitude of the recipients towards the donor could be a major contributing factor (Zargooshi

---

108 Rohter L. The organ trade: A global black market; tracking the sale of a kidney on a path of poverty and hope. New York Times. Published May 23, 2004.

109 Laino C. Going abroad for transplants has risks. WebMD Medical News [online]. Accessed September 27, 2007.

2001). It may be that the poor donor may be hoping not only to improve his financial position but also elevate his social standing in the eyes of the recipient. But in reality, the negative behavior of the more affluent and socially elevated recipient just serves to reinforce the donor's lowly social status further contributing to his emotional issues (Baines and Jindal 2003).

Despite the act of donation having being viewed as a business transaction, there still appears to be a stigma attached to organ donation with one study suggesting that 94 percent of the donors were unwilling to identify themselves as donors, even to close relatives (Zargooshi 2001).

Commercialization of organs in developing countries works against the philosophy in developed countries of organs being allocated on the basis of medical need[110]. However, despite medical need not being compatible with the rules of commercialization, the long wait for kidneys in developed countries is often a motivating factor in prompting these patients to travel to developing countries for transplants. In short, the commercialization of kidneys is feeding into the negative socio-economic issues prevalent in developing countries.

According to surveys compiled by the Coalition for Organ-Failure Solutions, which combats the trafficking of human organs, 48 to 86 percent of kidney donors in Egypt, Iran, India and the Philippines reported a deterioration in their health, such as being tired more easily and not being able to carry heavy loads as before[111].

While the arguments for and against a free market for kidneys is unavoidable and continues (Spital 2007), the first step, in our view, could be the establishment of a database in the Western countries of patients who have obtained their kidneys through commercial transaction. This could lead to identification of centers where these kidneys were obtained. A database would also identify surgical, medical and immunosuppressive protocols for recipients and donors in these hospitals. Another step would be to create a better liaison between the recipient and donor hospitals so that modern surgical and medical practices can be implemented. There should also be improved emotional and psychological support to both the recipient

---

110 World Health Organization: Guiding principles on human organ transplantation. Lancet 1991;337:1470.

111 Coalition for organ-failure solutions. http://www.cofs.org/what.htm

and the donor (Sajjad 2007; Joseph 2003). However, establishment of a database, may perhaps lead to an erroneous impression the academic community is condoning this practice.

The recent scandal in which a number of physicians in India were arrested while in the process of forcibly removing kidneys from poor donors for recipients from the Western countries suggest that this practice is still wide-spread and may represent just the tip of iceberg [112] [113]. But as long as the vast majority of people in Asia oppose donating their organs upon their death, black markets in poor countries where impoverished people sell their organs, especially kidneys, are likely to flourish[114].

Would a regulated market in kidney be the solution? An eminent Nephrologist, Dr. Eli Friedman, Distinguished Professor, SUNY-Downstate has made a case for a regulated market "Establishing a national regulatory council to coordinate and regulate marketed kidneys would be a logical extension of the present end-stage renal disease network collaborating with UNOS and OPTN. Eliminating black-market brokers would divert funds to actual kidney donors. Also, money saved from decreasing the number of prevalent dialysis patients might conceivably generate the total funding for additional kidney transplants. Positive points and main objections to legalizing living donor kidney marketing have been thoroughly analyzed. Before rejecting the concept of allowing kidney sales, it is helpful to consider those who are dying because of unavailable donor kidneys and might benefit from innovative thinking and fresh approaches."

Friedman goes on to compute the cost of a kidney in the regulated market "Nobel Laureate in economics Gary S. Becker and his colleague Julio J. Elias computed a 'market price' terming a live donor kidney a commodity. Assuming an American earning a mean salary of $40,000 annually (i.e., a life valued at $3 million), a 1 percent risk of death from nephrectomy, a 5 percent decrease in quality of life, and loss of $7,000 in income due to convalescence from surgery, appropriate compensation for that potential donors kidney would be $45,000. Using a more

---

112 Twilight trade. http://www.hindustantimes.com/special-news-report/TheKidneyScam/Twilight-trade/Article3-272424.aspx

113 Kidney thefts shock India. http://www.nytimes.com/2008/01/30/world/asia/30kidney.html

114 Demand soars on kidney transplant market. http://archive.newsmax.com/archives/articles/2007/4/3/143617.shtml

probable death risk of one in 3,000 nephrectomies (the reported risk is three in 10,000) reduces the kidney price to $20,000.[115]

CONCLUSION

Shimazono carried out a detailed survey on behalf of the Clinical Procedure Unit of World Health Organization (WHO)'s Department of Essential Health Technologies, which suggested that the international organ trade no longer represents sporadic instances in transplant medicine. He estimated that the total number of recipients who underwent commercial organ transplants overseas may be conservatively estimated at around 5 percent of all recipients in 2005. Moreover, undergoing transplantation through the international organ trade has become the most common way of undergoing organ transplantation in certain countries[116]. The WHO is of the opinion that there is an urgent need for further medical and social scientific research. The paucity of previous efforts to monitor the international organ trade arguably indicates an inadequate current mechanism to deal effectively with this global issue. Establishing a platform on which researchers, policy-makers, professional societies and international governing bodies cooperate in gathering and sharing information may be considered an essential step towards a more substantial international health policy[117]. Despite, a number of recent position statements position statements on transplant tourism voices have been raised that they are conceptually flawed. They have argued that the West is increasingly finding it fashionable to impose itself on the East with paternalistic and often self-serving policies that developing countries should conform to Western concept of ethics, socio-political and cultural beliefs, which, in turn, has become increasingly intolerant, overtly imperialistic and unacceptably antagonistic. It has also been known that transplant physicians from developing countries may support the commercialization of transplantation, are reluctant to voice

---

115 http://www.renalandurologynews.com/Marketing-Donor-Kidneys-A-Personal-Viewpoint/article/120102/

116 http://www.who.int/bulletin/volumes/85/12/06-039370/en/

117 *Resolution on human organ and tissue transplantation.* Geneva: WHO; 2004 (WHA 57.18). Available at: http://www.who.int/transplantation/en/A57_R18-en.pdf

their opinions out of fear that they will be ostracized by the transplant community[118].

A bill that could have made the law against organ trade ineffective in Pakistan has been withdrawn. The bill had proposed five amendments, including permission for donation to foreigners, a practice that had earned the country the notoriety of being an 'organ bazaar'. The proposed amendment had sought a 10 percent quota for donations to foreigners in medical emergencies. The amendments were opposed on the grounds that transplantations were not emergency procedures and the suggested changes would envisage commercial dealings and promote financial deals between buyers and sellers of human organs. It is of concern to note that 2,000 transplants had been carried out in the country and 1,500 of the recipients were foreigners. Over fifteen months since the promulgation of the law in September 2007, about 800 transplants have been done, of which 96 percent were related donations, four percent unrelated and 0.25 percent cadaver[119].

Nancy Scheper-Hughes[120] reported in Newsweek that illegal trade in human kidneys was being carried out in some of the top hospitals in the US. She has devoted a great deal of her professional life in tracking the illegal sale of human organs across the globe. She has proof that for approximately $150,000 per transplant, organ brokers can arrange for transplants in "broker-friendly" hospitals in the US. She claims in her report that brokers posed as or hired clergy to accompany their clients into the hospital and ensure that the process went smoothly. To summarize in the words of Frank Delmonico, from Harvard Medical School, Boston, US, and adviser to the WHO "Organ selling has become a global problem, and it's likely to get much worse unless we confront the challenges of policing it."

---

118 Am J Transplant 2008;8:1089.
119 http://dawn.com/2009/01/12/top14.htm
120 http://www.newsweek.com/id/178873/page/1

PROLOGUE

Chapter 17:
The Future of Kidney Transplantation in Guyana

International cooperation: To draw the peoples of the world together takes various forms, ours is one such attempt. Other agencies are also working in helping the developing world in bringing renal replacement therapies to their people. An innovative program has been undertaken by *Etablissement français des greffes* [121], which has been collaborating with a number of developing countries and East European countries. These programs have been aimed at supporting the development of procurement and transplantation programs, within a proper ethical and regulatory framework, tailored to the public health needs of each country. The main programs concerned Morocco, Tunisia, Romania, Bulgaria and to a smaller extent, Mexico and Vietnam. The main focus of these exchanges is to foster transfer of "know-how" between institutions and to improve cooperation amongst professionals within their hospitals and developing policies in the field of renal failure and kidney transplantation. The major drawbacks according to the French experience was reliance on a few highly motivated individuals, less satisfactory results in the projects aimed at developing procurement from deceased donors. Most of these organ transplantation programs rely on living donors: while this option is clearly relevant in terms of feasibility in particular, it is soon limiting and cannot alone provide access for all patients in need of an organ.

World Kidney Day: In an effort to increase awareness, detection, prevention, and treatment of kidney and related diseases, a "World Kidney Day" was established[122]. This effort aims to raise awareness <u>about the heavy</u> burden of chronic kidney disease (CKD) on

121 http://sysnews.multimodo.com/compoweb/590/file/Luciolli.pdf
122 www.worldkidneyday.org

human lives and health care budgets and put CKD on the agenda of governments and other institutions around the world that shape and reform health policy. This initiative assumes importance as recently published studies have confirmed that CKD is a more common disorder than previously thought. Clinical trials have recommended two simple and inexpensive tests are available to detect CKD: (i) urine for protein and (ii) blood for serum creatinine and hence estimated (iii) glomerular filtration rate (GFR). It seems that despite the availability and validity of this approach, the task of developing widespread detection and management programs for CKD that produce improved outcomes at a reasonable cost is formidable. It is unlikely that even developed countries have adequate financial and human resources for whole-population screening programs for CKD, and there is no clear evidence that these measures are cost-effective.

Based on current information, Shah and Feehally[123] on behalf of the World Kidney Day Steering Committee have recommended that all countries have targeted screening programs.

Steps to establishing an effective program include:
- Report of estimated GFR by all laboratories measuring serum creatinine.
- Measurement of eGFR and proteinuria in people at highest risk of CKD, including all those with diabetes, hypertension, coronary heart disease and cerebrovascular disease who constitute the majority of patients with CKD and with end-stage renal disease.
- Regular measurement of blood pressure, eGFR, and proteinuria in people identified with CKD.
- Establishment of targets for blood pressure control in people with CKD, and appropriate use of drugs blocking the renin-angiotensin system.
- Agreement on guidelines for identifying the minority of people with CKD who benefit from the specialist advice of a Nephrologist as well as the routine care of a family physician.

Suggested strategy for management of kidney failure in Guyana: There is a need for a Government-supported program for the large expanding end stage renal failure population. Simultaneously efforts should be

123 http://www.worldkidneyday.org/UserFiles/File/editorial08.pdf

made to plan and initiate a prevention/control program for CKD. To pick up CKD at an early stage, steps should be initiated to promote methodology for standardization and estimation of GFR rather than serum creatinine in clinical laboratories. Such data would prompt and enable physicians to pick up CKD at an earlier stage, improve the opportunity for early referral of CKD patients to Nephrologistss to minimize progression of CKD. Training of physicians to take care of patients with renal failure should also be undertaken and a national registry and prevention program should be undertaken as a matter of urgency. Kidney transplant program should be enhanced, as this is more cost-effective than dialysis. Long-term care of transplant patients should include the provision of subsidized medications.

More patients with renal failure being evaluated for kidney transplant: During our visits to Guyana, we screened five patients of whom three were found suitable for kidney transplant. We are communicating with the local physicians to work up these patients as shown in some e-mail exchanges below.

RE: Case note & pictures of possible patients

From: rahul jindal
Sent: Tue 9/09/08 3:15 PM
To: Anita Cumbermack; Ravi, Asha Purohit; Ramsundar Doobay; Khan, Michael; ministerofhealth
Cc: Kamela Bemaul; Ryhan Singh

Dear Anita:

I am summarizing the work up so far. Some tests need to be done ASAP, in particular for the first 3 patients and their donors.

1. Mr W G's work up is complete. His (MG) donor needs PAP smear, mammogram, second FBS and stool examination.

2. Ms N Y needs HB, FBS, Mammogram, PAP smear. Her donor (MN) needs mammogram, PAP smear, US

of the native kidneys, second FBS, urine culture and stool examination.

3. Mr T S needs Mantoux test, stool exam, FBS, PSA, VDRL and EKG. His donor (TS) needs mammogram, PAP smear, EKG, FBS, VDRL, urine and stool exam and PPD.

4. Mr P C and his donor (RW) are totally incomplete and need all the investigations.

Once, these tests are complete, you can proceed with the renal angiogram. We will not operate till all the tests are complete.

Please let me know when the tests are done so that I can send the tubes for HLA and cross-match.

Thank you,
Rahul M. Jindal, MD, PhD, MBA

Appeals to fund kidney transplants in Guyana: Guyanese newspapers are full of appeals for help in raising money to take patients to India or other countries for kidney transplantation. Mangal Munesh received a successful kidney transplant; however, many patients are still in need for transplants. We are planning more trips to undertake this procedure. Below are some of the appeals for help in a variety of medical conditions, however, it seems that kidney transplantation is the major cause for patients appealing for help[124.]

> Georgetown, Guyana, November 29, 2007: Kids First Fund is again appealing for public help as its major sponsor left the organization US$50,000 in debt after failing to make payments to the Frontier Lifeline Hospital at Chennai in India.
>
> Even as the organization struggles to make the payments, the state-owned vehicle that was loaned to the former First Lady, Mrs Varshnie Jagdeo, now Ms Singh, has since been taken back.

124 http://www.caribvoice.org/Pop%20Ups/help.html

Thus, Ms Singh launched an appeal, yesterday, to anyone from the public who owns a spare vehicle to loan it to the Kids First Fund for a few weeks.

At a press conference hosted at the National Communications Network (NCN) studio, Ms Singh revealed that the Ministry of Health never gave the promised airfare to the children.

According to her, after returning from the United States on September 28 last, where an appeal for help was launched, she received a phone call from the Ministry of Health.

She said she was told that the Ministry will pay for those children under the age of 18, but up until the departure date, no money was forthcoming.

The children have since undergone their surgeries and have returned with a second chance to live, Ms Singh said yesterday.

She, however, noted that she is still hopeful that the Health Ministry will make those payments.

The hospital bill in India totaled US$65,596 but the Kids First Fund was given a US$10,000 discount.

Unless the outstanding total is paid, children can no longer be taken for surgery at that institution.

Some 275 children are on the Kids First Fund's waiting list for surgery, she added.

Anyone wishing to make a donation to the organization can make contributions to account number 39415 at Scotia Bank, or 7332 at the New Building Society.

Annandale cancer patient needs urgent assistance

Annandale, Guyana, November 26, 2007: WHILE most married couples his age are enjoying family life, 24-year-old Mahendra Lall, who has been diagnosed with colon cancer, has been deprived of this comfort.

Lall's wife, Rovena Moharoop 20, in an interview with the Guyana Chronicle related that her husband, whom she met and married seven years ago, has been diagnosed with the deadly disease just over a year ago.

The grieving housewife who resides with her husband at 91, Gale St. Annandale, East Coast Demerara who is appealing for assistance from the business community and public spirited citizens said since.

Mahendra's grave illness was detected he has not shown any sign of recovery.

However, like most dedicated wives Rovena expressed optimism that her husband would recover, despite the fact that Guyana Cancer Institute has listed his condition as (stage iv B) or very critical.

The mother of three children, two girls and one boy told this newspaper apart from her husband's recovery, she is hoping that Housing Minister Harrynarine Nawbatt would pay heed to her house lot application.

Rovena, said she had applied about three months ago but on a recent visit to enquire about the state of affairs with her application was told by an official at the Housing Ministry that it has to be examined by the minister, which is expected to be done soon. Mrs. Lall is also calling for Human Service Minister Priya Manickchand's help for public assistance noting that to bring up her children has been an extremely tough task since her husband has been bed ridden. She said her husband, a former salesman at Survival Supermarket was the sole breadwinner of their household. His three children are Geetangale Lall, age six, Kashani age five and Kamish, one year and six months. According to Mrs. Lall, Geetangale is presently in grade one while Kashani is in her second year at nursery school. Meanwhile, the housewife expressed gratitude to Edward Beharry Group of Companies, Beacon Foundation and the public for their kind support in their difficult circumstance.

Documents from the Guyana Cancer Institute showed Lall has been recommended to take six cycles of 5-fluorouracil + Leucovorin Chemotherapy treatment. The institute which has also certified him for financial assistance said he has completed three of the cycles so far.

Persons interested in assisting the Lall's family can do so by making a deposit of any amount at the Demerara Bank on Account number 1218718 or Republic Bank on Account number 1760362.

Mother of two in dire need of kidney transplant

Guyana, November 4, 2007: Almost 14 months after being diagnosed with kidney failure, family members and close friends of 45-year-old Nazlima Mahamad, of 215 Lusignan West, East Coast Demerara, is soliciting monetary assistance form the general public in aid of her kidney transplant surgery in Pakistan.

After receiving prolonged treatment from the local dialysis centre for almost one year, Mahamad had sought alternative medical attention in India at the Colombia Asia Hospital.

Leaving for India around August this year, Mahamad was immediately admitted to the hospital but after more than two months on the waiting list, she was reportedly discharged since the hospital was somehow forced to abort the scheduled operation.

Acting on information provided by close family, friends and doctors, Mahamad has begun the pursuit of yet another avenue, this time in Pakistan. Though this avenue is evidently more reliable than the other, the price attached is surprisingly much more than the family has anticipated - an estimated US$20,000. Not deterred by this sum, the Mahamad family is driven by quest to their mother in their lives. Raising about US$5000 thus far through telethons and contributions from Kaieteur News Publisher Glenn Lall and owner of Guyana Stores Limited Tony Yassin, the family has received a boost but is still lagging by about US$15,000. As such, they are seeking the assistance of the general populace. Mahamad was diagnosed around mid September last year, when she started experiencing severe swelling in both her legs, and was admitted to the Balwant Singh Hospital. Subsequent to the admission, the family was reportedly informed that both of the woman's kidneys had ceased to function, and she required immediate dialysis treatment.

This treatment was started in a Trinidadian hospital, but due to the high costs was continued in Guyana to the tune of approximately $37,000 per treatment, which was required about three times per week. A telethon was held as recent as last Friday on MTV Channel 65, by the woman's 19-year-old daughter Wazlima Mahamad, where the family managed to raise approximately $700,000 in pledges and has so far collected roughly $500,000. Another telethon is carded for tomorrow on NTN Channel 69 from 20:30 hrs to 22:30hrs.

Persons interested in making monetary contributions and those interested in finding out more about the woman's condition can contact telephone numbers 627-5927, 696-0000, 695-2235, 686-5247, and 696-8888.

Those interested in making contributions through the bank can do so at the Demerara Bank Limited to account number 1220391.

Nazlima Mahamad is currently in Pakistan with her son who is handling the financial and other arrangements, as she awaits her kidney transplant surgery.

Young mother appeals for help for dialysis treatment

Guyana September 14th 2007: Twenty-nine-year-old Reena Sultan is appealing to the public to assist her with the cost of dialysis treatment, which she needs urgently.

When Reena suddenly collapsed seven years ago and was rushed to hospital she and her family were given the devastating news that her kidneys were failing. Since then life had progressed fairly okay as she went to the clinic, got medication and was able to care for her husband and son.

Two months ago her life changed again when she took a turn for the worse as the condition of her kidneys deteriorated. The young mother is now wheel-chair bound, and gets exhausted easily. Reena's husband of eight years, Fazil, who was working as a computer technician, quit his job to help her.

Fazil told Stabroek News on Tuesday that his wife's condition was diagnosed as chronic renal failure and because of its progression she needs dialysis treatment urgently. Dialysis is a medical procedure that uses a machine to filter waste products from the bloodstream and restore the blood's normal constituents, a function which a healthy kidney performs. He said that Reena had been in and out of hospital recently and that her condition is deteriorating. Fazil said over the past months he has been going around seeking help as the cost of treatment is expensive.

Fazil said that the cost of the initial treatment is $215, 000 then his wife would need to access the treatment twice per week at a cost of $36, 050 per session. Fazil said his wife needs the treatment urgently. "She needs to be on dialysis," he declared. The couple is appealing for help in accessing the treatment.

Fazil said that the Ministry of Health has pledged to fund 10 of the dialysis sessions but he would have to do the rest. He also said that he has looked at the cost of a kidney transplant and the Apollo Hospital in New Delhi, India had quoted a price of US$18,500 for a ten-day stay in the hospital, the surgery and medication.

He said that for now, his wife urgently needs the dialysis as her condition is worsening. "It's getting so severe, I don't want it to end up at the stage when she could collapse and leave me," he said.

Anyone willing to help the couple can call 683-9861 or 227-4167 or can donate directly to their Citizens Bank account number 218334826.

Mother of two needs $3M for urgent renal transplant

Georgetown, Guyana, June 4, 2007: A 26-year-old mother of two, battling end stage renal failure (ESRF) has less than two weeks to raise an additional $3M desperately needed to meet the overall bill of $6M for her to have a kidney transplant done in India by mid month, in order to save her life.

Deokawattie Bharrat of Conservancy Dam, Canal Number 2, West Bank Demerara, and her relatives are hoping and praying in earnest that the corporate community and other civic minded persons can continue to chip in to help make it possible for her to have this life saving surgical intervention. Unless this is done, the young mother, now facing a grim future, must be prepared to continue to pay the cost of about $.75 million per month for her to continue living on dialysis.

Four years ago, Deokawattie who fell from the top of a stairway when she was just four years old, was diagnosed with chronic renal failure. An ultra sound of the abdomen at 22, revealed that she had bilateral shrunken kidneys. That condition, according to her doctors "has now degenerated into ESRD, and is in need of urgent renal replacement therapy", meaning that both her kidneys have shut down, and she needs to have a kidney transplant done without delay.

Whilst finding a replacement for a damaged kidney is no easy task, Deokawattie has already found a donor her 27-year-old sister, Rookmin Dilip who also lives at the Boerasirie Conservancy Dam.

Rookmin, out of love for her sister, even after having been counseled and briefed on the implications for the donor, has willingly agreed to give up one of her kidneys in order to save the life of her younger sister. She has already had all the necessary tests done, and has been rated as a safe and compatible donor for Deokawattie.

Account numbers given are: GBTI: 51BB573953 and Republic Bank: 765-493-2.

'I am begging Jamaica to help my daughter'

Kingston, Jamaica, May 24, 2007: A few months ago she was a regular bubbly student, who was eager to learn and enjoyed playing with friends.

Today, nine-year-old Danielle Harriott, who was diagnosed with bone marrow aplasia, a condition which makes her prone to life-threatening bleeding, is unable to walk and do the things that once made her happy.

As a result of her condition, Danielle is anemic; she bleeds through her nose and eyes, gets high fever and is unable to speak properly. Danielle's condition is difficult to treat and the treatment is not available locally. As such, her mother, Cassandra Christopher, is making an urgent plea to the nation to assist her daughter who is desperately in need of surgery, which will cost about J$6 million.

Currently unemployed: The public has already given the family $400,000 but Ms. Christopher, who is currently unemployed as a result of her daughter's condition, believes that through this medium, the public may dig deeper into their pockets to assist. Her daughter was diagnosed with the illness in March and has since been hospitalized at the Bustamante Hospital for Children.

"I am begging Jamaica to help my daughter to do this surgery so she can come home because every time she says she wants to come home," said Ms. Christopher.

"The other day mi drop down because mi can believe this would happen to mi daughter," said a tearful Ms. Christopher, adding that every time she passes Danielle's school - Dunrobin Primary - she cries.

Ms. Christopher, who spends most nights and days with her daughter at the hospital, says Danielle is very worried about her illness.

"The other day she asked, if she go to sleep if she will wake up," said Ms. Christopher.

The eldest of four children, Danielle helps her 31-year-old mother to read. Persons who would like to assist her, can make payments to Danielle Harriott, Jamaica National Building Society account number 10588930.

Trini in Canada appeals for kidney

Toronto, March 25, 2007: After trying three years to find a suitable kidney donor, 36-year-old Nalini Maharaj is hoping to have success in Trinidad and Tobago - the land of her birth.

Maharaj, originally from Couva, has been living in Mississauga, Canada, for the past 14 years with her husband Puran and two children ages 18 and 20. She began experiencing renal failure in both kidneys ten years ago and lost kidney function in 2003. She has been going for dialysis three times a week.

In an interview with Sunday Newsday from her home in Canada, Maharaj said she is trying to find a donor in TT because for the last three years she has been on a waiting list and her condition has recently worsened. "I am trying because the waiting time is much longer (in Canada). Plus it would be easier to get a match (in TT)," she said. Her blood type is AB.

Maharaj's renal failure occurred because of high blood pressure. This chronic disease and diabetes runs in her family and eliminates them as donors. Her husband cannot donate as he has high blood pressure. She said donors must be "healthy enough to donate."

She expects to get a "transplant" quicker in Trinidad than wait for years in Canada. Newspaper advertisements highlight her appeal.

She is an auditor with a plastic company. "It is hard to work because of tiredness. It affects your entire family, everything—the stress."

She said people who are willing to assist can contact her via email at puran8@msn.com. Earlier this month, Health Minister John Rahael launched the National Organ Donor Programme at Crowne Plaza. He said the donor program would bring relief to people who have end stage renal failure and approximately 400 people were having dialysis at public health facilities.

He said there were "several unlisted others" who "in a couple of months" would experience kidney failure.

The donor program recently started a sensitization program about donating kidneys and corneas.

Nine kidney transplant surgeries took place last year under the national organ transplant program.

Dhanrajh's life of pain: Man needs US$90,000 for liver transplant

September 4th 2006, Port of Spain, T&T: First he had restless nights. Then upset stomachs and severe abdominal pains. And then he started vomiting blood. Before he fell ill, Dhanrajh Persad had frequented the gym and had led a fairly active lifestyle, so that when he suddenly got sick, he could not understand why - neither could his parents. Dhanrajh was first hospitalized at the Sangre Grande Hospital and was later transferred by ambulance to the Port-of-Spain General Hospital, where he underwent more medical examination as doctors tried to determine what was wrong with him. The results were not good; he was diagnosed with cirrhosis of the liver of unknown etiology.

Cirrhosis of the liver is characterized by hardening of the liver as a result of damage to the liver cells over years. It can ultimately lead to liver failure. The disease is most commonly caused by excessive intake of alcohol, but Dhanrajh knew to himself that he never abused alcohol and would only drink occasionally, like around Christmas time, so he was taken aback with his diagnosis.

Doctors informed him that the damage to his liver could not be reversed or treated and his only option was to have a liver transplant, which may help prolong his life. In the months following, Dhanrajh began losing weight, dropping from 187 pounds to 123 pounds. He now experiences severe back pains, severe cramps and abdominal pains and still has restless, sleepless nights. His illness forced him to change his diet and lifestyle completely -no salty or spicy foods, no meat, no curry, eat lots of vegetables, his doctor advised him.

Dhanrajh spends up to $800 monthly for various medications he must take on a daily basis, which among other things, helps him to pass out fluid that his body retains and "thins" his blood so that it does not clot and cause complications. He feels exhausted all the time and cannot walk or do anything without feeling tired. His illness has also forced him to lay off his job as an estate constable. He is currently on extended sick leave. However, the liver transplant he must undergo and which would likely help him to lead a normal life again would cost approximately US$90,000 - money he and his family do not have. The procedure is to be done at a transplant centre in Argentina.

From since 2004, the year he was diagnosed with his condition, Dhanrajh and his close relatives have embarked on several fund-raising ventures. Although being considerably successful, the ventures have brought them nowhere near the US$90,000 figure. Dhanrajh, 34, is now appealing to the public to help him raise the funds so he can undergo his operation in the soonest possible time. "We are still a long way off from the target," he told the Express. "There are a lot of people who have contributed so far and we appreciate it very much but we still need help. I'm asking if you all can help us raise this money."

He said he has already found a donor and it was now left up to his family to raise the necessary funds. My brother has the same blood type and he has agreed to give me a portion of his liver. What we have to do now is get the money. The doctor told me that based on condition of my liver; they are giving it about two years. I'm almost to the end of the second year. The doctor said I should try and get the operation done before the liver gets worst.

Dhanrajh, a resident of Sangre Grande, said he believes that once his operation was successful he would be able to lead a normal life again. He said young Akil Wilson, who was diagnosed with cirrhosis and portal hypertension of the liver last year and was now healthy and doing well after undergoing his liver transplant operation in Argentina last year, have also given him renewed hope. "Seeing him alive has given me hope. When he left here he was in a real bad condition and to see that he went and get his transplant done and is now back and doing well, he is an inspiration to me," Dhanrajh said.

Akil had shot into the spotlight last year after his mother, Sharon Wilson, a housewife, came forward with a public plea for help to raise $3 million so he could undergo the life-saving transplant operation in Argentina.

Dhanrajh said that he had kept his fingers "crossed" for Akil when he learned that he was finally able to go to Argentina for his operation. The Universitario Austral Hospital in Argentina, which his family had located, had agreed to treat him and defer payment of US$300,000 for the operation. "I thought to myself that if his surgery was successful, then maybe mine could be successful as well," Dhanrajh said. "I kept my fingers crossed for him and when he pulled through I felt happy for him and for myself."

Dhanrajh's mother and father, who had accompanied him to Express House, Port of Spain, said they wanted nothing more than to see their son back to his old self again. "He was so very active," Leela Persad said of her son, the eldest of four children. "He was always in gym. He would go camping and fishing but most of the things he used to do he can't do them anymore," she said. "It is not easy seeing him in this condition. I myself have sleepless nights. I shed a lot of tears behind closed doors because I don't want him to see me crying because I know it will bring him down. We love him and we want him to have a full life. I would be so happy if he gets his operations but we really need the help to raise the money."

Dhanrajh's father, Parmanan, said the family has had to foot the cost for his son's medical bills and this was quite challenging. He also said that the drugs his son uses were not covered under Government's Chronic Disease Assistant Programme (CDAP).

In the interim, the younger Dhanrajh longs for a proper night sleep. He says since falling ill he continues to have restless, sleepless nights. "I always feel so exhausted but still I can't sleep properly. I am awake at all hours in the night. When I think I'm resting I get up and still feel tired. Walking from there to here will tire me out."

Dhanrajh said he wants to be himself again and feels the public could help make this happen by donating funds which would help him pay for his life-saving liver transplant operation.

Lisa needs our help
Lisa Stephen is in need of a kidney transplant, after suffering from kidney failure

Port of Spain, T & T: An urgent plea has come from family members and close friends of a young woman of Morne Road, Castries who is now living in dire straits. Twenty-two-year-old Lisa Stephen is in need of a kidney transplant, after suffering from kidney failure. Stephen, a past student of the St Joseph's Convent and the Sir Arthur Lewis Community College (SALCC) Division of Arts and General Studies (DASGS) was diagnosed with her ailment in 1999. At the time, she was still a student and it never stopped her from continuing her studies-finishing the DASGS program in honors.

Loved ones describe Stephen as a fighter and have now turned to the public for whatever assistance they can give. Lisa's struggle continues to increase as her health worsens. Presently, calcium deposits have rendered her immobile and she has been restricted to her home since January this year. Her mother has been helping in whatever way she can, carrying to Stephen her dialysis treatments three times a week.

Stephen's circumstances have hindered her working life and this has come at a great loss to her as she was the only breadwinner in her household.

She waits hoping that donations from the public will assist in covering the cost of her US$100,000 medical surgery and intervention. All donations to this cause can be made to account number 414242 at the Bank of Nova Scotia in Trinidad & Tobago.

Chapter 18:

Second Kidney Transplant Carried Out and More to Be Carried Out

Two kidney transplants in New Year[125]

December 25, 2008, By KNEWS
New dialysis centers to be opened

In the first quarter of 2009, two more kidney transplants are to be conducted in Guyana. At a press conference held yesterday at the Ministry of Health, Health Minister Dr. Leslie Ramsammy said that the doctors have already made their preparations; testing has been completed, and the persons are now being brought together.

The first kidney transplant was done in Guyana in July, and it was deemed successful. Munesh Mangal, 18, of Lusignan, East Coast Demerara, who had for many years suffered from renal failure, received a kidney from his mother, 41-year-old Leelkumarie Nirananjan Mangal. And Minister Ramsammy said that two new dialysis centers will be introduced in 2009, which will significantly reduce the burden on the 5G Dialysis Centre.

---

125 http://www.kaieteurnews.com/2008/12/25/two-kidney-transplants-in-new-year/

One of the new centers will be opened next month, and the other, which would be run by the Central Islamic Organization of Guyana (CIOG), will come on stream not much later. According to Dr. Ramsammy, with the introduction of these dialysis centers, it will be cheaper by half for people to access dialysis.

"So that will make dialysis more comprehensively available in Guyana. At the moment, virtually everyone who goes to 5G needs to seek our help," Dr. Ramsammy said. However, although there will be two additional centers in the country, it will still not significantly reduce the number of people going overseas for transplants.

The ministry will be spending some $100 million on the medical assistance program which helps persons to get medical care, some of which is not available in the public health system. Now many of these medical interventions are now being offered in Guyana.

Dr. Ramsammy explained that some of the money will now be spent in Guyana. Previously, all the money was spent predominantly on persons seeking medical attention abroad. According to Minister Ramsammy, heart conditions are the number one reason why persons seek assistance overseas. He explained that, of the $100 million, 27 percent went to people with heart diseases. A further 13 percent went to cancer victims. Money also goes to treating kidney diseases, surgery, dialysis and transplants.

Love moves kidney donor – Second kidney transplant carried out successfully[126]

By Stabroek staff On February 5, 2009

---

126 http://www.stabroeknews.com/news/love-moves-kidney-donor/

Just for love Melissa George decided to give one of her kidneys to her ailing father last week Sunday and if she had to make the decision again she would not hesitate.

Speaking to Stabroek News last evening from the High Dependency Unit (HDU) of the Georgetown Public Hospital (GPHC), the 25-year-old immigration officer said that her father, Winston George, is the best father in the world and "love does not have to motivate anyone."

She was moved from the Intensive Care Unit (ICU), where she was with her father since Sunday after the transplant, to the HDU and she was happy with reports that she would more than likely go home today. The young woman said she is feeling "very good except for a little pain in my side."

She described her father as being like a friend with whom she can discuss anything. "We would sit down and talk, have family time.

He is the best father anyone could have," the young woman said from her hospital bed. She said that she was the one who took the decision to give her father a kidney even though he was somewhat hesitant. When the first transplant was done here she showed him the newspaper report and told him it could have been him. She and a sister then took it upon themselves to get the test done and her kidneys were a match and she did not hesitate to sign up to make the donation to her father. She said on the day of the transplant she was not afraid nor did she ponder about any post-transplant pain as the only thing on her mind was giving her father a longer lease on life.

"I am only now praying that everything goes well and he is home soon and well," the young woman said.

And her mother, Loraine George, expressed gratitude to the overseas team for the successful operation and also thanked the Minister of Health, Dr. Leslie Ramsammy for facilitating the operation.

She said her husband is now sitting up and eating by himself and brushing his teeth but he cannot leave his bed at the moment. "He is eating anything. He said the doctor told him to eat up and he asked me for bake and sausage," the woman said last evening

George, an ex-army major, was diagnosed with renal failure since in 2000 and on Sunday he became the second person in local medical history to receive a kidney transplant. The first transplant was done seven months ago and Sunday's operation on the 47-year-old man was done in record time since the foreign doctors were more familiar with the local operating theatre.

George, who served the army for 17 years before he was sent off as medically unfit, was placed on peritoneal dialysis since 2000 but was told that after a period of ten years he would have to obtain a kidney transplant.

However, last year the man became very sick suffering from stomach pains and vomiting constantly. He had to be placed on the haemofiltration dialysis, but yet he was in and out of the Georgetown Hospital where he had joined the kidney clinic. It was while at the clinic he met with the foreign team and was later identified as a likely candidate.

The operation, which was led by US transplant surgeon Dr. Rahul Jindal, commenced at around 8 am on Sunday, 1st February, 2009 and was completed around 1.30 pm.

The overseas medical team that performed the operation included the Indian-born Dr. Jindal of Brookdale University Hospital; Dr. Eduard Falta, Transplant Surgeon of the Walter Reed Army Medical Center (WRAMC), Washington; Dr. Melanie Guerero, Pulmonary Care Physician; Laura Owens, Transplant Coordinator; and Dr. Arthur Womble who is attached to the Athens-Limestone Hospital, Athens, Alabama. (Oluatoyin Alleyne)

Second kidney transplant recipient talks about his pre-transplant challenges[127]

February 8, 2009 – By KNews

Nine years ago, when Winston George was diagnosed with renal failure, his life took a turn he never catered for. Two years after being diagnosed, George, who became the nation's second kidney transplant recipient at the Georgetown Public Hospital, was deemed medically unfit to serve in the Guyana Defense Force, and was forced to resign, after dedicating some 22 years of his life to the army. It was not so easy letting go of something he loved so much; nevertheless, George said, he had to give up his job and, before long, as a result of his deteriorating condition, his childhood dream, too, was shattered.

According to George, during his final year at the University of Guyana, while studying to become an Agriculturist, he was forced to give up his studies to seek overseas treament.

"What was more heartrending was not being able to work and to provide for my family…I remember one morning I began to cry because it really hurt knowing I have children to provide for, and at that time my wife was not working," George recalled. As if losing

---

127 http://www.kaieteurnews.com/2009/02/08/second-kidney-transplant-recipient-talks-about-his-pre-transplant-challenges/

his job and having to deal with his illness was not enough, giving up his studies just compounded the situation.

"I always wanted to become an Agriculturist; and after giving up my job and having to leave my studies, it was not easy." Nevertheless, like the Biblical character Job, George never gave up on himself or his family. While having to deal with dialysis, George said, being surrounded by family members and loved ones who were all supportive kept him going. Throughout his illness, George said, the most difficult part was to leave his children behind to seek treatment in Barbados, where he was a total stranger and had no one else but his wife and God to depend on.

"When we arrived in Barbados, I was in the hospital on treatment and my wife and my sister were there with me in the initial stages. Then I received tremendous help from the then Major-General of the army, Joe Singh."

As time went by, the cost for treatment became more and more expensive, and hope of survival was getting bleaker, George said. "The turning point for me was one day I met a young man who was only 19. He was suffering from the same illness, and I was talking with him in his hospital bed. During our conversation, he just died," George recalled. At that point, George said, he knew he had to do something more about his illness, and he immediately began finding out what his options were. As the years progressed, George said, it was brought to his attention that having a kidney transplant was an option and would give him a few more years of being with his family.

"When I first found out about kidney transplant, I joined the clinic at the Georgetown Public Hospital; and after seeing that a transplant was done successfully here, I began considering that," George said. According to George, not knowing if he would be eligible for the transplant, he and his family began making preparations. "We just start doing all the tests to find a donor, and initially my brother said he was going to be the donor; then he subsequently pulled out," he recalled. At that point, my two daughters opted to be donors, but I at first disagreed.

"I recalled when my two eldest daughters said they were willing and I told a friend, and his words to me were, 'Boy, let those girls have their lives'."

After thinking long and hard, George said, he was still hesitant, but his eldest daughter, Melissa, insisted; and with her persistence, George said, he finally agreed. However, while the family was preparing, they had not yet contacted the Ministry of Health to see if he was eligible. George said that he penned a letter to the Minister of Health, and within a matter of two days he got a response. "It was amazing. The Friday I sent the letter and the Monday morning the Minister's Secretary called, and I was told to visit the Georgetown Public Hospital. And before we knew it, they asked us if we could find a donor, and that we should start doing a series of tests," George recalled.

Fortunately for George and his family, they had already completed most of what was required of them. As the time drew near for the surgery, George said, he was a bit worried, but he managed to draw courage from his daughter who donated the kidney.

"At times I was getting cold feet, but I knew I had to stay strong for her, and I did just that…even up to the day of the surgery I was a bit worried, and what compounded the situation was something Melissa did before she was going into the operating room"

"When the doctors were wheeling Melissa into the theatre, she raised herself up from the stretcher and waved at me…Right away I remembered that that was the same thing Dr. Cheddi did when they were wheeling him onto the airplane days before he died," George said amidst tears.

However, after seeing the reassuring smile on his daughter's face, George said, he immediately dispelled all negative thoughts from his mind. Like his daughter, the last thing he recalled before going into surgery was being prayed for by the doctors. Once the surgery was over and he regained consciousness, George said, his first question to the doctor was, "Where is my daughter?" After he was reassured that both he and his daughter were doing well and the surgery was successfully completed, he said, he cried again. Now that both George and his daughter have passed what they deemed as the worst part, and they are both back home in the care of their family, their focus is now on getting back to normal lives. George said he is seriously considering going back to the University of Guyana to complete his studies. To his daughter for her life-saving gesture, George said "To me, I knew I did my best for my children, but I never thought my best was to their standard and what they were looking for." To his wife, George said, he is thankful to her for not giving up on him. "Throughout this ordeal, I was able to see a side of my wife I never saw in all the years we were together. I know she is a tower of strength," George said. With a radiant smile, George also expressed his gratitude to the Ministry of Health, the staff at the Georgetown Public Hospital, and other overseas experts who performed the surgery.

The kidney transplant, the second to be performed locally, was completed in record time at the Georgetown Public Hospital last Sunday, and George was discharged on Friday while his daughter was sent home on Thursday. The surgery was done by Dr. Rahul Jindal, who was aided by his overseas team as well as local health personnel.

The first kidney transplant was conducted last August.

Even minor problems become news!
Kidney transplant patients given requisite care at GPHC – Dr. Purohit[128]

March 30, 2009, By kaieteurnews

Kidney transplant patients are afforded after-care services at the Georgetown Public Hospital Corporation that has proven to be on par with services offered at other medical facilities outside of Guyana.

This is the view of Dr. Ravi Purohit, a surgeon who has had direct involvement with the two kidney transplant operations that were undertaken here last year and last month respectively under the leadership of India-born doctor, Rahul Jindal.

Dr. Purohit's declaration came in response to questions about the capabilities of the local facility to adequately render follow-up care in wake of reports that the most recent kidney recipient, former Army Major Winston George was re-admitted to hospital with concerns about his health.

George had received a kidney from his 25-year-old daughter, Melissa George, an Immigration Officer.

The operation was successful and both patients were discharged within a matter of days. However, George was readmitted to the public institution last Tuesday after he became concerned about his health.

---

128 http://www.kaieteurnews.com/2009/03/30/kidney-transplant-patients-given-requisite-care-at-gphc-%e2%80%93-dr-purohit/

The 47-year-old man, who was accompanied to the hospital by his wife, Lorraine, had disclosed that he was feeling weak and was hardly able to eat solid foods. He was also experiencing a burning sensation.

Speaking from his bed in the High Dependency Unit of the hospital, George, who was being administered saline, related that it was since the previous week that he had told his doctor about his condition. He said that he was advised by the doctor to return to the hospital at anytime if the condition persists.

At that time George claimed that his main concern was the fact that he seems to be consuming more water than the doctor recommended.

He had attributed his weakness to the fact that he has not been eating much solid foods and his general health was been dampened by the burning sensation in his mouth, which had persisted for some time since his operation on February 1.

George said he was informed that the burning sensation is in fact a side effect of the operation and should have been appeased by the use of a mouthwash, which was provided by the hospital.

However he was later told that because he did not utilize the mouthwash in the correct way he had developed a fungus in his mouth, which is responsible for the burning sensation in his mouth.

His condition has since improved although he is now faced with concerns about his blood sugar level.

But according to Dr. Purohit, who has responsibility for George's aftercare, the fungal infection (Candida) that George has contracted is not uncommon in transplant patients.

According to Dr. Purohit, with the utilization of the available treatment at the hospital, George will be better in a few days and it is expected that he would be discharged soon after.

The Wikipedia free online encyclopedia states that "Candida is a genus of yeasts. Clinically, the most significant member of the genus is Candida albicans, which can cause infections (called candidiasis or thrush) in humans and other animals, especially in immune-compromised patients.

"Transplant patients take medications to suppress their immune system as an anti-rejection measure, as do some patients suffering from an over-active immune system."

Health Minister Dr. Leslie Ramsammy has said that the onus still remains on kidney transplant patients to also take responsibility for their recovery.

At a press conference held prior to George's operation, the Health Minister related, "It is not only up to the doctor and how good a job they do but it is also up to patients, who also have a major responsibility. We can take care of them and provide all the things they need but if they do not take care of themselves they will not heal as fast. They must take their medication because that is something we cannot do for them."

According to the Minister the issue of follow-up must be emphasized as important to patients since it should be a rigid responsibility, which is in fact critical to their recovery.

"When the operation on transplant patients is finished, how well they do will be dependent on how well they and their family follow instructions," Minister Ramsammy asserted.

He also disclosed that even after Dr. Jindal and his team leave Guyana, they continue to assist the local experts to monitor the patients.

"They do not disengage themselves from the patients. We are always talking with them and we do telemedicine conferences so in fact, they never walk away."

Additionally, the Minister noted that the patients of the first transplant never stopped gaining the medical attention of the foreign doctors.

On July 12th last year 18-year-old Munesh Mangal of Lusignan, East Coast Demerara, received a kidney from his 41-year-old mother Leelkumarie Nirananjan Mangal. They are both said to be doing well.

Chapter 19:

Politics As Usual Even In Medical Charities

Disenchanted With the Ministry of Health in Guyana-Prominent Philanthropist Turns his Sights on Education[129]

February 18, 2009 - BY DR. TARA SINGH

The much anticipated 2nd kidney transplant was conducted at the Public Hospital Georgetown Corporation (PHGC) on January 30, 2009 by a US-led medical team headed by Dr. Rahul Jindal and Dr. Edward Falta. The recipient was former Army Major, Winston George, 47, and the donor was his daughter, Melissa George. Both father and daughter are showing good signs of recovery. Dr. Jindal had also headed the medical team that conducted the 1st kidney transplant in the country on Munesh Mangal, 17 on July 12, 2008. Shortly after Winston George's surgery, Guyana's Minister of Health, announced to the nation and the world that the 2nd kidney transplant was a success. But we, as observers, must never allow the New York based pioneers of this project to go unnoticed, either. It was a non-medical person, Mr George Subraj, together with his Coordinator Mr Lake Persaud, as well as, his New York associates, who broke the proverbial ice

129 http://www.thewestindiannews.com/?s=Disenchanted+With+the+Ministry+o f+Health+in+Guyana-Prominent+Philanthropist+Turns+his+Sights+on+Educ ation

and set in motion the right atmosphere for kidney transplants to take place in Guyana. While others, including medical personnel, were skeptical whether such an operation could be successfully performed in Guyana, the US project leader George Subraj had always been optimistic about the outcome. Apart from the significant role played by the medical team, including Dr. Arthur Womble, we also compliment the following NY team members: Mr Tony Subraj, Mr Jaskaran Persaud, and Mr Kawall Totaram. But success always tends to breed its own enemies. There appeared to have been some kind of conflict in the role and expectation between the New York team and the Ministry of Health. We know, for example, that a regular complaint of the Ministry has been that overseas medical teams tend to interfere with the country's medical policies and protocols. For his part, George Subraj and his associates vehemently rejected this charge. "We respect existing medical policies and protocols, and never attempted to subvert these. All we seek was medical help for needy patients by providing the expertise and resources. We leave the observance of medical protocols to the medical personnel.

Our main task is to put together the team, manage the logistics, such as traveling, accommodation, and publicity, and provide the resources." Lake Persaud notes: "We also ensure that proper after care is provided to patients, including the pursuit of rehabilitative services." For the benefit of readers, it would be recalled that the 2nd kidney transplant surgery, as well as, three others was supposed to have been facilitated by George Subraj and his New York associates, but that did not happen. Instead, it seemed that the Ministry of Health pulled the rug under their feet when they engaged in direct negotiations with the US medical team, without any input from George and his colleagues. The New York team had anticipated that ugly development and sought a meeting with the Minister of Health to work out any differences. Four members of the New York team traveled to Guyana in November 2008 to meet with the Minister to discuss the plan for the 2nd kidney transplant, among other things. To avoid future conflicts, the Minister agreed to issue, within a few days, the New York team with a letter of understanding (LOU) setting out their expected role and function in this process. The New York team left that meeting feeling that everything was back on track. However, after several weeks passed by, and they did not receive the LOU from the Ministry of Health, they began to feel uneasy. All attempts to get further information on the second kidney transplant project were frustrated.

George and Lake decided to have an audience with the President who was passing through New York on his way to Libya. The President assured them that their efforts are appreciated by the Guyana government and encouraged them to continue with the kidney transplant project, even if they have to recruit a new medical team. So, they persevered. The New York team is baffled why they were excluded from the 2nd kidney transplant project since they had an understanding with the Ministry that they would serve as "facilitators" of the kidney project. To unravel, therefore, what had become a mystery to them, George Subraj, Lake Persaud, and Anand Rambharose traveled to Guyana in late January 2009, which happened to coincide with the 2nd kidney transplant surgery there. They received a cold reception from the authorities, and their attempts to have an official meeting with the Ministry of Health did not materialize, either. Despite their humiliation, they were warmly received by the medical team, and they even invited them to lunch. The NY team asked itself, "How could we serve as facilitators when they didn't provide us with such basic information on the size of the medical team and how long they will stay in Guyana, as well as, the scheduled date of the operation."

The New York team just want some respect. After all, they were the ones to help set the pioneering kidney transplant surgery into motion at a heavy personal and financial cost of over $30,000. While other groups had taken patients to India for kidney transplant, George thought that it would be a better idea to take the doctors down to Guyana where they could also train local medical personnel to conduct such surgeries in the future; a process that could add sunlight into the lives of hundreds of Guyanese and their families. When asked about their exclusion, George Subraj and Lake Persaud believe that it might relate partly to the question of control, turf battle, and the possible infusion of financial incentives for the medical team that had apparently been negotiated between the Ministry and an international bank. The announcement following the 2nd kidney transplant surgery that the medical team plans to conduct one such operation every three months, further reinforced their belief in the role of financial incentives. Let's hope that the welfare of patients remains the dominant consideration, and that it does not become a casualty of the monetary incentive.

But the dynamic New York philanthropist, Mr George Subraj, vowed to continue with his mission of helping the needy. While his promise of conducting four more kidney transplant surgeries may not materialize in the present environment, that prospect is not strong enough to stifle his passion for humanitarian work. Hundreds of groups eagerly seek George's benevolence. Thus, he is currently building a $60,000 state-of-the-art Computer Laboratory at Swami Aksharananda's Saraswati Vidya Niketan High School. The Lab will be equipped with 50 computers, a security system, and necessary infrastructure, and is scheduled to open in August 2009. He is helping to modernize the Hindu Temple at Bel Air, Georgetown, as well as, donating the tiling to the newly constructed Mora Point, Mahaicony Health Clinc. And in New York, he came to the assistance of the Prem Bhakti Mandir of Jamaica, Queens, by donating the $(US)36,000 elevator to this elegant $(US)600,000 monument. Not to mention his patronage of several cultural events, including the annual Holi Sammelan Progam of March 14, 2009. Despite his disenchantment with developments in the kidney transplant project of Guyana, George Subraj and his NY team's commitment to medical outreach will never falter.

George's and Lake's impact will be felt through the famous Guyana Watch (GWI) organization, in which George serves as Vice President. The work of George Subraj, as well as, his business, Zara Realty Corp, is well known in New York, Toronto, Guyana, and elsewhere. Our community has become better because of their remarkable philanthropic work. We commend George and his colleagues for their resilience, and for their struggle to help Guyanese and others

Written by The West Indian

Comments
5 Responses to "Disenchanted With the Ministry of Health in Guyana-Prominent Philanthropist Turns his Sights on Education"

James on February 19th, 2009 9:01 pm
George Subraj is a slum landlord. He is well known for seeking publicity and cheating his tennants. Please don't give us this nonsense about Subraj doing Guyanese people any favors. Ask anyone in Queens,

NYC, and they will tell you that Subraj is a slum landlord.

Andrew on February 19th, 2009 9:03 pm
I agree with James. It is good that the Ministry of Health has stood up to Subraj and his family. They have exploited the Guyanese community for too long. Shame on you Subraj.

Ram on February 19th, 2009 9:20 pm
George Subraj should stop paying reporters to plant these one sided stories. Dr. Tara Singh did not bother to contact the Minister of Health or the patients. I think the article was written by one of Subraj's cronies and placed here by paying some money. It is called "yellow journalism".

Shree on February 22nd, 2009 2:54 pm
I am disgusted by George Subraj who is planting stories by a discredited writer. Tara Singh should stop taking money from Subraj to write this nonsense. Guyanese people should celebrate about the progress made in our country and take our country to a higher level.

Great job by GPHC, Minister of Health, local doctors and the foreign team.

Chamcha on February 22nd, 2009 9:09 pm
Dr Tara Singh - you are an expert at yellow journalism. You bring a bad name to all journalists. Zara Realty is known for its strong arm tactics and bad behavior. Ask any Guyanese in Queens or Liberty Av in New York City.

Some things are just not right at GPHC[130]

July 20, 2008, By Knews

---

130 http://www.kaieteurnews.com/2008/07/20/some-things-are-just-not-right-at-gphc/

Within recent times, there have been many complaints about the operations of the Georgetown Public Hospital. The most recent complaint was leveled by a woman who gave birth to a baby that was said to have been stillborn.

This woman claimed that she never saw her baby because she was under an anesthetic. She said that when she recovered no one could tell her anything about the baby. Weeks later, after the woman went to the press and her predicament became public knowledge, the hospital duly went public with the fact that the baby was in the mortuary of the hospital.

If this is the case, then something had to be wrong. The woman must have been visited by relatives who would have asked about the baby. Certainly, the persons who asked must have not got any response, and being simple people, they would have muttered and moved on.

We argue that the hospital should have informed the mother instead of waiting until she went public. Another issue involved a young girl who died because the hospital failed to diagnose her ailment, and in the end the girl died.

The child's mother said that she took her daughter to the hospital with pains, and after a brief period of observation the hospital gave the girl some medication and sent her home. A few days later, the child was rushed back to the hospital, and again there was nothing more to be had than some tablets. By the time the hospital recognized that something was seriously wrong, the girl was dead. She had succumbed to a ruptured appendix.

A week ago, there was this former officer of the Customs Anti-Narcotics Unit who was discharged from the hospital having been taken there suffering from hypertension. The man died a few hours later at home.

We have had people who went to the hospital for hysterectomy and died, some hemorrhaging because the surgeons could not stop the bleeding. And in one case a woman died because she was given aspirin although she was allergic.

The problem seems to be the shortage of skilled medical practitioners at a time when the administration is boasting about providing a vastly improved service. The hospital is performing a series of new surgeries, the most recent being a kidney transplant.

The hospital is also supposed to be doing hip replacements and heart surgeries. Any facility that can do such things should be able to diagnose ailments. Indeed, many ailments could present the same symptoms, so that further investigation is necessary. This seems not to be the case at the Georgetown Public Hospital.

But for all this, the hospital has scored many successes largely because visiting doctors are coming home to share their skills and, as some say, to give back to the society. Some crucial surgeries have been performed, and the locals have had a chance to work with these visiting experts.

The problem, however, is that the locals often do not have the chance to practice what they have learnt, because on their own they simply cannot undertake the program.

There is therefore the need for the experts. In Guyana, these experts are the consultants, who are spread thin because they often lend their services to the private hospitals.

So we come back to the problem of missed diagnoses, a situation that could mean life or death. We know that the staff at the Accident and Emergency Unit is hard pressed, given the number of cases the few doctors and the nurses have to see each day.

One is led to believe that, because of the pressure of work, the doctors are not paying enough attention to the people seeking medical attention. Perhaps this is why the man was sent home to die, and why the young girl died of a ruptured appendix.

Dr. Leslie Ramsammy is making a lot of noise about the number of doctors coming back from Cuba. One can only hope that they undergo a successful period of internship and that they actually learnt their trade over the period that they were in Cuba.

It would not be unreasonable to conclude that many people died because enough attention was not paid to them. Just this past week, people who were seeking medical attention at the Georgetown Public Hospital opted to seek the services of the visiting doctors who are here as part of Guyana Watch. They claim that these doctors find their complaints while the locals cannot.

The same thing happened when the Americans brought a medical ship off the Guyana coast.

REFERENCES

Abbey S, Farrow S. Group therapy and organ transplantation. Int J Group Psychotherapy 1998; 48:163.

Ai AL, Peterson C, Bolling SF. Psychological recovery from coronary bypass graft surgery: the use of complementary therapies. J Alt Compl Med 1997; 3:343.

Alexander GC, Sehgal AR. Barriers to cadaveric renal transplantation among blacks, women, and the poor. JAMA 1998; 280:1148.

Arici M, Altun B, Usalan C, et al. Compliance in hemodialysis patients: unanticipated monitoring of biochemical indices. Blood Purif 1998; 16:275.

Auer J. Social and psychological issues of end-stage renal failure. In: Parsons FM, Ogg CS, eds. Renal failure – Who cares? Lancaster: MTP Press, 1983.

Baines LS, Jindal RM. Non-compliance in patients receiving haemodialysis: an in-depth review. Nephron 2000; 85:1.

Baines LS, Joseph JT, Jindal RM. Compliance and late acute rejection after kidney transplantation: a psycho-medical perspective. Clin Transplant 2002; 16:69.

Baines LS, Jindal RM. Non-compliance amongst kidney transplant patients: a psychosocial perspective. Transplant Proc 2001; 33:1900.

Baines LS, Jindal RM. Consequences of selling kidneys in India. JAMA 2003; 289:697-700.

Burnham T, Phelan J. Mean Genes. Middlesex: Penguin Books Ltd, 2001.

Bame SI, Petersen N, Wray NP. Variation in hemodialysis patient compliance according to demographic characteristics. Soc Sci Med 1993; 37:1035.

Bernardini J, Piraino B. Compliance in CAPD and CCPD patients as measured by supply inventories during home visits. Am J Kidney Dis 1998; 31:101.

Blake CW, Courts NF. Coping strategies and styles of hemodialysis patients by gender including commentary by Porter L and Gurkis J, with author response. ANNA Journal 1996; 25:477.

Botting D, Review of the literature on the effectiveness of reflexology. Compl Ther Nurs Midwifery 1998; 6:10.

Bramstedt KA, Xu J. Checklist: Passport, Plane Ticket, Organ Transplant. Am J Transplant 2007; 7:1698-1701.

Ben Hamida F, Ben Abdallah T, Goucha R, et al: Outcome of living-unrelated (commercial) renal transplantation: report of 20 cases. Transplant Proc 2001; 33: 2660–2661.

Chiang W, Chung H. Hemodialysis patient's fatigue relating to depression, social support, and blood biochemical data. Nur Res China 1997; 5:115.

Christensen AJ, Moran PJ, Lawton WJ, et al. Monitoring attentional style and medical regimen adherence in hemodialysis patients. Health Psychology 1997; 16:256.

Courts NF. Stress inoculation education and counselling with patients on hemodialysis: Effects on psychosocial stressors and adherence, PhD thesis, University of North Carolina, 1991.

Cramer JA. Practical issues in medication compliance. Transplant Proc 1999; 31:21.

Cramer JA. Relation between medication compliance and medical outcomes. Am J Health Syst Pharm 1995; 52 [Suppl. 3]:27.

Craven J, Farrow S. Surviving Transplantation. University of Toronto Press, 1993.

Cvengros JA, Christensen AJ, Lawton WJ: The role of perceived control and preference for control in adherence to a chronic medical regime. Ann Behav Med 27:155,2004.

Covic A, Seica A, Gusbeth-Tatomir P et al: Illness representations and quality of life scores in hemodialysis patients. Nephrol Dial Transplant 19:2078,2004.

Chugh KS, Jha V. Commerce in transplantation in third world countries. Kidney Int 1996; 49:1181-1186.

Canales MT, Kasiske BL, Rosenberg ME. Transplant tourism: Outcomes of United States residents who undergo kidney transplantation overseas. Transplantation 2006; 82:1658-61.

DeOreo PB. Hemodialysis patient-assessed functional health status predicts continued survival, hospitalisation, and dialysis-attendance compliance. Am J Kidney Dis 1997; 30:204.

Drummond-Young M, LeGris J, Brown G, et al. Interaction styles of out-patients with poor adjustment to chronic illness receiving problem solving counselling Soc Work Health Care 1996; 4:317.

Diaz-Buxo JA, Lowie EG, Lew NL, et al. Quality of life evaluation using Short Form comparison in hemodialysis and peritoneal dialysis patients. American Journal of Kidney Diseases 35:293, 2000

Davidson AM. Commercialization in organ donation. Nephrol Dial Transplant 1994; 9:348-349.

Furr LA. Psycho-social aspects of serious renal disease and dialysis: a review of the literature. Soc Work Health Care 1998; 27:97.

Frishberg Y, Feinstein S, Drukker A. Living unrelated (commercial) renal transplantation in children. J Am Soc Nephrol 1998; 9:1100-3.

Ghods AJ, Savaj S Iranian model of paid and regulated living-unrelated kidney donation. Clin J Am Soc Nephrol 2006;1:1136-45.

Goyal M, Mehta RL, Schneiderman LJ, Sehgal AR. Economic and health consequences of selling a kidney in India. JAMA 2002; 288:1589-93.

Goetzmann L, Klaghofer R, Spindler A et al: The Medication Experience Scale for Immunosuppressants (MESI): initial results for a new screening instrument in transplant medicine. Psychother Psychosom Med Psychol 56:49,2006.

Howells N, Maher EJ. Complementary therapists and cancer patient care: developing a regional network to promote co-operation, collaboration, education and patient choice. Eur J Cancer Care 1998; 7:129.

Haq I, Zainulabdin F, Naqvi A, et al. Psychosocial aspects of dialysis and renal transplant. J Pak Med Assoc 41:99, 1991.

Higgins R, West N, Fletcher S, Stein A, Lam F, Kashi H. Kidney transplantation in patients traveling from the UK to India or Pakistan. Nephrol Dial Transplant 2003; 18:851-2.

Hussein MM, Mooij JM, Roujouleh H, el-Sayed H. Commercial living nonrelated renal transplantation: observations on early complications. Transplant Proc 1996; 28: 1941–1944.

Inston NG, Gill D, Al-Hakim A, Ready AR. Living paid organ transplantation results in unacceptably high recipient morbidity and mortality. Transplant Proc 2005; 37:560-2.

Ivanovski N, Popov Z, Cakalaroski K, Masin J, Spasovski G, Zafirovska K. Living-unrelated (paid) renal transplantation - Ten years later. Transplant Proc 2005; 37:563-4.

Ivanovski N, Stojkovski L, Cakalaroski K, Polenakovic M. Living unrelated (paid) renal transplantation: besides the ethics. Transplant Proc 1997; 29:3631.

Jindal RM, Joseph JT, Morris MC: Noncompliance after kidney transplantation: A systematic review. Transplant Proc 35:2868,2003.

Joseph JT, Baines LS, Morris MC, Jindal RM. Quality of life after kidney and pancreas transplantation: a review. Am J Kidney Dis 2003; 42:431-45.

Katayama F, Kodama M. Effect of nursing counselling on acceptance of hemodialysis treatment in elderly women patients. Jpn J Counsell Sci 1994; 27:53.

Kahan K. Psychiatric considerations. In: Kahan BD, Ponticelli C, eds. Principles and practice of renal transplantation. London: Martin Dunitz Ltd, 2000.

Kimmel PL, Thamer M, Richard CM et al: Psychiatric illness in patients with end-stage renal disease. Am J Med 105:214,1998.

Kandel P. India: The kidney bazaar. Lancet 1991; 337:1534.

Leggat JE Jr, Orzol SM, Hulbert-Shearon TE, et al. Non-compliance in hemodialysis: predictors and survival analysis. Am J Kidney Dis 1998; 32:139.

Latham CE. Obstacles to achieving adequate dialysis dose: compliance, education, transportation, and reimbursement. Am J Kidney Dis 1998; 32 [Suppl. 4]:93.

Lopes AA, Bragg J, Young E et al: Depression as a predictor of mortality and hospitalization among hemodialysis patients in the United States and Europe. Kidney Int 62:199, 2002.

Montemuro M, Martin LS, Jacobsen S, et al. Participatory control in chronic hospital based hemodialysis patients including commentary by Brunt JH, with author response. ANNA J 1994: 21:429.

McDade-Montez EA, Christenen AJ, Cvengros JA et al: The role of depression symptoms in dialysis withdrawal. Health Psycho 25:198,2006.

Morad Z, Lim TO. Outcome of overseas kidney transplantation in Malaysia. Transplant Proc 2000; 32:1485-6.

Mansy H, Khalil A, Aly TF, et al. Outcome of commercial renal transplantation: two years follow-up. Nephron 1996; 74:613-6.

Naqvi SA, Ali B, Mazhar F, Zafar MN, Rizvi SA.A socioeconomic survey of kidney vendors in Pakistan. Transpl Int 2007.

Overbeck I, Bartels M, Decker O et al: Changes in quality of life after renal transplantation. Transplant Proc 37:1618,2005.

Prasad GV, Shukla A, Huang M, D'A Honey RJ, Zaltzman JS. Outcomes of commercial renal transplantation: a Canadian experience. Transplantation 2006; 82:1130-5.

Procci WR: A comparison of psychosocial disability in males undergoing maintenance hemodialysis or following cadaver transplant. Gen Hosp Psychiatry 2:255, 1980.

Power RE, Hayanga AJ, Little DM et al: Outcome of cadaveric renal transplantation in patients with psychiatric disorders. Ir Med J. 95:172,2002.

Perez-San-Gregorio MA, Martin—Rodriguez A, Galan-Rodriquez A et al: Psychologic stages in renal transplant. Transplantation Proceedings 37:1449,2005.

Sciarini P, Dungan JM. A holistic protocol for management of fluid volume excess in hemodialysis patients. ANNA Journal 1996; 23:299.

Sensky C, Leger C, Gilmour S. Psychosocial and cognitive factors associated with adherence to dietary and fluid restriction regimens by people of chronic hemodialysis. Psychother Psychosom 1996; 65:36.

Skotzko CE, Stowe JA, Wright C, Kendall K, Dew M. Approaching a concensus: Psychosocial support services for solid organ transplantation programs. Progress in Transplantation 2001; 11:163.

Sensky T: Psychiatric morbidity in renal transplantation. Psychother Psychosom 52:41,1989.

Schlebusch L, Pillay BJ, Louw J. Depression and self-report disclosure after live related donor and cadaver renal transplants. S Africa Med J. 75:490, 1989.

Sanfey H, Haussman G, Isaacs I, et al. Steroid withdrawal in kidney transplant recipients: is it a safe option? Clin Transplant 11:500,1997.

Sun CY, Lee CC, Chang CT, Hung CC, Wu MS. Commercial cadaveric renal transplant: an ethical rather than medical issue. Clin Transplant 2006; 20:340-5.

Spital A, Taylor JS. Living organ donation: always ethically complex. Clin J Am Soc Nephrol 2007; 2:203-4.

Sajjad I, Baines LS, Salifu M, Jindal RM. The dynamics of recipient-donor relationships in living kidney transplantation. Am J Kidney Dis 2007; 50:834-54.

Teran-Escandon D, Ruiz-Ornelas J, Estrada-Castillo JG, et al. Anxiety and depression amongst renal transplantation candidates: impact of donor availability. Actas EspPsiquiatr 29:91, 2001.

Thiagarajan CM, Reddy KC, Shunmugasundaram R, et al. The practice of unconventional renal transplantation (UCRT) at a single center in India. Transplant Proc 1990; 22:912-914.

Vlaminck H, Maes B, Jacobs A, Reyntjens S, Evers G. The dialysis diet and fluid non-adherence questionnaire: validity testing of a self-report instrument for clinical practice. J Clin Nurse 2001; 10:707.

Wiebe JS, Christensen AJ. Health beliefs, personality, and adherence in hemodialysis patients: an interactional perspective. Ann Behav Med 1997; 19:30.

Watnick S, Kirwin P, Mahnensmith R et al: The prevalence and treatment of depression amongst patients starting dialysis. The American Journal of Kidney Disease 41:105,2003.

Walsh D. Transplant tourists flock to Pakistan, where poverty and lack of regulation fuel trade in human organs. The Guardian [online]. Accessed September 27, 2007.

Yeh TL, Huang CL, Yang YK et al: The adjustment to illness in patients with generalized anxiety disorder is poorer than in patients with end-stage renal disease. Journal of Psychosomatic Research 57:165, 2004.

Zargooshi J. Quality of life of Iranian kidney "donors". J Urol 2001; 166:1790-9.

Zargooshi J. Iranian kidney donors: motivations and relations with recipients. J Urol 2001; 165:386-92.